T0021301

LACTIVATE!

LACTIVATE!

A USER'S GUIDE TO BREASTFEEDING

JILL KRAUSE

AND

CHRISIE ROSENTHAL, IBCLC

ILLUSTRATION BY ANGELICA YIACOUPIS

ROCKRIDGE
PRESS

Copyright © 2019 Rockridge Press, Emeryville, California

No part of this publication may be reproduced, stored in a retrieval system, or trans-mitted in any form or by any means, electronic, mechanical, photocopying, recording, scanning, or otherwise, except as permitted under Sections 107 or 108 of the 1976 United States Copyright Act, without the prior written permission of the Publisher. Requests to the Publisher for permission should be addressed to the Permissions Department, Rockridge Press, 6005 Shellmound Street, Suite 175, Emeryville, CA 94608.

Limit of Liability/Disclaimer of Warranty: The Publisher and the author make no repre-sentations or warranties with respect to the accuracy or completeness of the contents of this work and specifically disclaim all warranties, including without limitation war-ranties of fitness for a particular purpose. No warranty may be created or extended by sales or promotional materials. The advice and strategies contained herein may not be suitable for every situation. This work is sold with the understanding that the Publisher is not engaged in rendering medical, legal, or other professional advice or services. If professional assistance is required, the services of a competent profes-sional person should be sought. Neither the Publisher nor the author shall be liable for damages arising herefrom. The fact that an individual, organization, or website is referred to in this work as a citation and/or potential source of further information does not mean that the author or the Publisher endorses the information the indi-vidual, organization, or website may provide or recommendations they/it may make. Further, readers should be aware that websites listed in this work may have changed or disappeared between when this work was written and when it is read.

For general information on our other products and services or to obtain technical support, please contact our Customer Care Department within the United States at (866) 744-2665, or outside the United States at (510) 253-0500.

Rockridge Press publishes its books in a variety of electronic and print formats. Some content that appears in print may not be available in electronic books, and vice versa.

TRADEMARKS: Rockridge Press and the Rockridge Press logo are trademarks or registered trademarks of Callisto Media Inc. and/or its affiliates, in the United States and other countries, and may not be used without written permission. All other trade-marks are the property of their respective owners. Rockridge Press is not associated with any product or vendor mentioned in this book.

Interior and Cover Designer: Tricia Jang
Art Producer: Sue Bischofberger
Editor: Morgan Shanahan
Production Manager: Riley Hoffman
Production Editor: Chris Gage
Illustration © 2019 Angelica Yiacoupi

ISBN: Print 978-1-64152-958-7 | Ebook 978-1-64152-959-4
R0

THIS BOOK IS DEDICATED TO
ALL PARENTS AND CAREGIVERS –
HOWEVER YOU CHOOSE
TO FEED YOUR BABY.
YOU'RE DOING A GREAT JOB!
—JILL KRAUSE & CHRISIE ROSENTHAL

CONTENTS

INTRODUCTION: HOW TO USE THIS BOOK

You've had breasts for a while. It's safe to assume you're pretty familiar with them, right? But when it comes to getting your breasts to perform the task of lactating and feeding your baby, it's not always simple.

Breastfeeding can be overwhelming and confusing for many of us, even those of us who have breastfed before. It may be "natural" but there's nothing wrong with you if you don't feel like it comes naturally.

The purpose of this book is to give you some quick references and resources to demystify breastfeeding and without bogging you down in the process. We know free time is scarce when you have a newborn and exhaustion can zap any ability to focus, so you'll find a lot of to-the-point information in here, coupled with easy-to-understand illustrations.

We also want to be sure that while you're doing the sometimes-hard work of learning (or relearning) how to breastfeed, you're also taking care of yourself. We've written this manual with your mental health in mind because we believe what matters most is a happy and healthy baby and mom.

Who are we and what makes us qualified to write this book?

I'm Jill Krause, and I have been breastfeeding my four babies for roughly 95 months and counting. I'm a parenting and pregnancy blogger, and I've connected with thousands of other moms over the last decade and listened to many of their stories of breastfeeding struggles and triumphs. I'm also passionate about guarding moms' mental health, and I have been open about my own personal battle with postpartum anxiety and OCD.

I've partnered with Chrisie Rosenthal, IBCLC, to write this book. Chrisie is a board-certified lactation consultant with three boys of her own, including a set of twins. She has 10 years of professional experience, including teaching hospital classes, running breastfeeding support groups, and partnering with families at the Land of Milk and Mommy, her Los Angeles–based private practice. Chrisie is all about evidence-based, judgment-free, practical advice that enables women to make the best decisions for themselves and their families.

We hope this book quickly becomes a valuable part of your parenting tool kit.

We will cover the basics, like:

- When should my milk come in?
- Why are my breasts so hard?
- Are pacifiers going to ruin everything?
- How will I know if this is working?

We'll also cover more specific topics, like:

- ◊ Can I try to conceive while breastfeeding?
- ◊ What happens to my lactating breasts when I have sex?
- ◊ Can I take my mental health medications while breastfeeding?
- ◊ What do I do if this is really painful?

We are not assuming breastfeeding will be challenging for you or that you'll fail. We're also not assuming it will be easy. Instead, we want to empower you and give you all the information you'll need to make breastfeeding work for you and your baby for as long as you feel like it's a good fit.

MOM TO MOM

"Have confidence. Nurse in the way that feels comfortable. In public. In private. Cover or no cover. Whatever makes you and baby feel comfortable. Have confidence in your body and its ability to feed your baby. Confidence to keep going when it's hard or you feel judged. It will be worth it. Just be confident and trust the process."

— Anna, Tule Lake, CA

FAQ

WILL BREASTFEEDING HURT?

Although it may be a little uncomfortable in the beginning, breastfeeding should not be painful or leave you with cracked, bleeding nipples. Some lucky moms experience no pain at all, but most new moms will feel a little tenderness in the beginning. The most common experience is to feel a little pinching or "tugging" when baby latches on, which quickly subsides. Good positioning and a deep latch are key to breastfeeding comfortably. If the latch hurts, make sure you ask your nurse, pediatrician, or lactation consultant for help right away.

WHEN WILL MY MILK COME IN?

For the first three to five days you'll have colostrum, which is highly specialized, concentrated milk that's meant for baby's first days. It's pretty magical! Colostrum acts as a laxative and helps stabilize your baby's blood sugar. A full meal is 5 to 10 milliliters, perfect for a newborn tummy, which is roughly the size of a cherry. Check out the visual on page 73. (Fun fact: Your breasts started making colostrum around week 14 of pregnancy!)

When your baby is around three to five days old, your milk will transition from colostrum to mature milk and your breasts will probably feel fuller. You may notice baby taking gulps of milk and see milk dripping from their mouth when they're done. Be sure to feed on demand. The more baby feeds, the more milk your body will make!

WHAT IF I'M UNCOMFORTABLE WITH THE IDEA OF BREASTFEEDING?

It's super normal to not know how you're going to feel about breastfeeding. You've never done this before, and there are a lot of unknowns. Most new moms don't realize it's going to be a learning process for you and for baby. Be patient and give yourself at least six weeks to get the hang of it. Remember, there's no one way to breastfeed. Breastfeeding may be all at breast, or it may involve pumping and bottle-feeding. Breastfeeding can also include formula supplementation.

WHAT IF I DON'T HAVE ENOUGH MILK?

Here's the good news: 90 percent of first-time moms have enough milk to feed their baby! Only 10 percent of moms have issues with low milk supply. Your pediatrician will be following your baby's weight gain and let you know how it's going. You should also track the number of feeds, pumps, sessions, and wet and dirty diapers each day and be ready to report those numbers at baby's checkup. If your pediatrician feels your baby needs to be supplemented with formula, they will let you know, and then you can reach out for help with your supply. Plans for boosting low supply vary and may include interventions such as increasing breastfeeding frequency, pumping, herbs, or prescription medication.

ARE THERE FOODS I CAN'T EAT?

Nope! Breastfeeding moms should eat a healthy, varied diet. Nothing is off limits. All those stories you hear about no spicy foods, no foods that cause gas, and no chocolate are myths. That includes foods that you were advised to avoid during pregnancy, too. Almost all babies will be fine with mom returning to a normal, healthy diet. Of course, take standard precautions to avoid food poisoning, because, well, it's no fun and getting dehydrated can reduce your milk supply. If you head to a sushi place, make sure it's high quality, and avoid anything old or suspicious in the fridge.

WILL FORMULA MAKE MY BABY SLEEP LONGER?

Here's the scoop: Formula does take longer for a baby's body to digest, so it will generally keep a baby full for a longer stretch of time. The reason it takes longer to digest is because formula is harder to break down. That can back-fire if your goal is longer sleep for baby. You may end up with a baby who has more gas, spit-up, or other uncom-fortable symptoms that keep them awake. And remember, if you want to keep up a full supply, you'll need to pump in place of the formula bottle. There are pros and cons to both breastfeeding and formula feeding.

WILL I EVER BE ABLE TO BREASTFEED IN PUBLIC?

Yes, but it's going to take time and practice. When you first learn to latch your baby, it will probably feel very method-ical. It may not be easy to latch quickly and casually, and that might leave you feeling somewhat "exposed." With time and practice (and the right clothes) breastfeeding will become much easier, and you'll get the hang of it. Pretty soon, you'll find that you're able to feed anywhere without giving it a second thought! If you can, bring a supportive partner or friend with you the first time you try breast-feeding in public. Do a trial run by choosing a public but comfortable spot, like a park bench. Latch baby while your support person looks out for you, if that makes you feel better. With practice, it gets easier!

WHEN CAN I START PUMPING AND BOTTLE-FEEDING?

As a general rule, between three and six weeks is the perfect time. By then, breastfeeding is established and baby can go back and forth between bottle and breast easily. However, sometimes we do need to use bottles earlier than three weeks. Whenever you give your baby a bottle, make sure you're using a slow-flow nipple, pouring an appropriate amount of milk into the bottle, and using the paced bottle-feeding method (see page 149).

DO I NEED A HUGE "STASH" OF BREAST MILK IN MY FREEZER?

Nope! If you're returning to work, you'll need about 20 to 30 ounces saved up. Most moms can start storing that about a month before their back-to-work date. If you're not returning to work, you only need enough for a few bottles. In fact, focusing on creating a stash can lead to overproduction and unnecessary stress. Remember to feed the baby, not the freezer!

WHAT BREASTFEEDING SUPPLIES DO I NEED?

All you *need* is your breasts and the baby. But we also recommend a good breastfeeding pillow (like My Brest Friend), a high-quality personal breast pump (it should be free from your medical insurance company), the Haakaa (a portable silicone hand pump), breast milk storage bags, an insulated/zippered lunch bag with a couple of frozen gel packs for breast milk transport, and a wrap for babywearing.

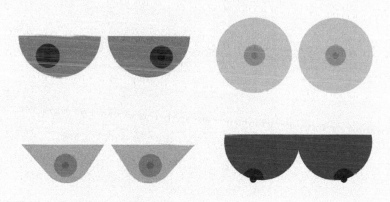

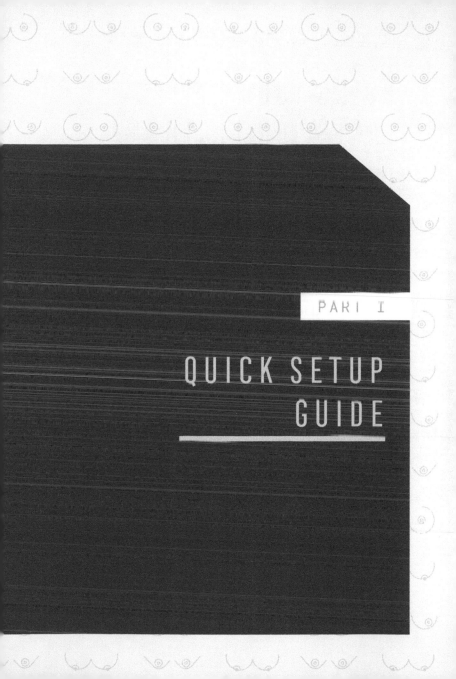

PART I

QUICK SETUP
GUIDE

USING YOUR NEW LACTATION FEATURE

MILK PRODUCTION

Breast milk is produced in highly specialized glands in your breast. When you breastfeed or pump, your body triggers those glands to release the milk and to make more milk. Think "demand and supply." If you are breastfeeding more than one baby, you'll be removing enough milk for multiple babies and that tells your body to produce more milk! Although your milk supply quickly ramps up in volume over the first few weeks, baby's average daily intake plateaus around week two or three at 25 ounces. That's good news because it means that you don't need to make more and more milk as baby gets older. (Phew!) The average breast milk bottle is 3 to 4 ounces at three weeks, and it stays that way the whole time. Your breast milk will continue to change to meet baby's growing needs, but the volume stays the same.

MILK RELEASE

The process of milk being released from the glands in your breasts is called "let-down."

Let-down can feel like:

◌ Pins and needles

◌ Electric shocks

◌ Tingling

◌ Itching

◌ A rush of milk

◌ Burning

◌ Sudden fullness

◌ Tickling

◌ Pressure

◌ Nothing at all

MILK TRANSFER

Attaching your baby to your breast is called "latching." When a baby latches, they typically suck rapidly to trigger the let-down response. Then baby will use a combination of suction, compression, and a wave-like motion of their tongue to remove milk from your breast. Your baby will transfer milk in bursts of sucking and swallowing. Once the pauses between bursts of sucking slow down and become farther apart, baby is done with their feed. The average breastfeed takes about 15 to 25 minutes total.

HEALTH CHECK: BABY BLUES VS. POSTPARTUM DEPRESSION

Following baby's arrival, mom will again experience major shifts in hormones that can lead to emotional swings. Sixty to 80 percent of moms report feeling the "baby blues," which typically last a few weeks and may look like unexpected bouts of sadness, anxiety, or irritability. Additionally, 8 to 20 percent of new moms in the United States experience postpartum depression and anxiety (PPD/A). PPD/A can appear anytime during pregnancy and up to one year postpartum according to the American College of Obstetricians and Gynecologists. While baby blues can look like sadness, mood swings, and frequent crying, moms experiencing postpartum depression and anxiety often feel overwhelmed and helpless. They may have trouble bonding with their baby or doubt their ability to care for their baby.

Did you know postpartum depression and postpartum anxiety are the leading complications from childbirth? Why aren't we talking about it more? There are many forms of help available, including therapy, support groups, and prescription medications. Contrary to popular belief, many medications are compatible with breastfeeding. Check out more about mental health on page 44.

MOM TO MOM

"If it's hard at first, don't give up! Find a breastfeeding support group in your area if it exists there. That support and understanding, plus the community, helped me and made me get out of the house!"

— Ana, Raleigh, NC

MILK DUCTS, LACTIVATE!

Around day three to five, your milk will change from colostrum to transitional milk. This is a hormonal process triggered by the delivery of your placenta during birth. Some moms will become engorged (super full) at this stage. We are talking breasts so big, so rock hard, so veiny, that they might feel foreign. It's wild, it's a little scary, and yes, it can definitely hurt. These boobs have a job to do now, though, and they are taking it very seriously. (This may also be about the time you tell your partner to never, ever touch them again. That's a normal reaction.)

Often, engorgement happens in the middle of the night. You may wake up to find yourself in a puddle of milk. That's super normal. (By the way, it's also normal if you don't get engorged. Some moms experience a more gradual transition.) If you find yourself uncomfortably engorged, do not use pumping or heat as your primary means of relieving engorgement. This will compound the issue, making your breasts fuller and more uncomfortable over time. Instead, apply cold compresses (bags of frozen peas or corn work great) to your breasts for 15 minutes a couple of times an hour, and continue to feed baby on demand. Avoid applying cold right before the feed. If you are so full that no milk will come out, then apply warm compresses right before the breastfeed for a few minutes. The initial engorgement should resolve in 24 to 48 hours. If it lasts longer, reach out to a lactation consultant.

MILK GLANDS

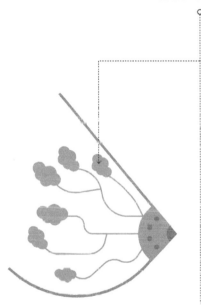
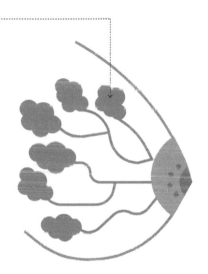

NOT ENGORGED:
The normal lactating breast is softer and mom is comfortable.

ENGORGED:
The engorged breast is full, hard, and sore. The pressure can cause damage to the cells.

STANDARD EQUIPMENT DIAGRAM

BREASTS: Mammary glands extending from the front of the chest, which produce milk in pubescent and adult females.

LOBULES: Glands where breast milk is produced.

DUCTS: Network of tubes that carry the breast milk from the lobules to the nipple.

AREOLA: Circle of darker skin around the nipple. It typically gets darker during pregnancy, which may be a visual clue to help baby find the breast.

MONTGOMERY GLANDS: Small glands around the areola (they look like little pimples!) that secrete a natural oil, which cleans and lubricates the nipple and areola. The oil also contains antibacterial properties to protect the breasts from infection, and it smells like amniotic fluid to help the baby find the breast. (Mother Nature is really giving baby lots of clues to find that breast!)

Lactocytes in mammary alveoli produce milk in response to sensory nerve inpulses.

Alveolus containing milk transport and lactiferous ducts

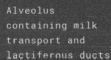

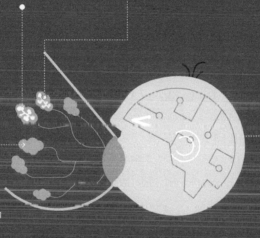

Mammary glands containing alveoli

Infant brain

Oxytocin triggers myoepithelial cells to squeeze milk from alveoli so it drains into lactiferous ducts.

Increased milk production triggers increased suckling by infant (positive feedback loop).

BREAST ACTIVATION DAY

Your body has never accomplished as much in one day as the day you gave birth. No matter how your baby exited your body or where you were when that happened, the biological machine that is you just succeeded in performing the impressive task of birthing a human (or humans). And it's not done yet. It's time to *LACTIVATE!*

The moments immediately following birth are crucial to setting your next programmed task—lactation—into motion.

Whether you give birth vaginally or via C-section, ideally your baby will be placed skin-to-skin on your chest immediately, if baby and mom are both healthy and stable.

The first hour of baby's life is also known as the "golden hour" and can be a very important time. It's ideal that mom and baby are not separated unless medically necessary. All measurements and observations can be done while you are holding your baby. If baby needs to be taken from you for anything, including a bath, request that it be put off for at least an hour.

Please know that if you missed out on the golden hour and immediate skin-to-skin contact, you are not destined to fail at breastfeeding—just feed as soon as you and baby are together again.

MOM TO MOM

"Don't compare yourself to other moms. You're all doing what's best and possible for your babies. As long as baby is fed, you're doing great!"

— Nikki, Ann Arbor, MI

BONDING POST-BIRTH

Bonding with baby is not one moment in time, but rather it's a continuous experience. If you didn't have the birth you planned for, or if you were separated from your baby, it doesn't mean that you won't have a meaningful bonding experience.

Skin-to-skin—laying baby on your chest so they can smell you, hear your heartbeat, and feel your warmth—is a very powerful way of bonding. If baby is already clean and bundled in blankets and a onesie, you can undress them and remove your top so that you can place them on your chest. Cover baby with a blanket if necessary.

At home, babywearing can be a great way to get in lots of skin-to-skin, keeping your baby happy and your arms free!

Some moms enjoy a "re-birthing bath" once they're both cleared to take a bath. This tends to be especially powerful for moms who didn't birth their baby or who didn't have the birth they planned for.

Recipe for a "re-birthing bath":

- Draw a shallow, lukewarm bath.
- Mom gets in the bath first.
- Either mom or a support person puts baby in the water on their back (being careful to keep baby's ears out the water).

- Mom or support person holds baby and allows baby to "float" in the water (this is meant to re-create the womb experience).

- Mom can talk to, sing to, or gently stroke baby.

- When baby is relaxed, place baby tummy down on mom's tummy in the water. Baby may crawl toward the breast and may latch and start breastfeeding.

BABY IN THE NICU

Your baby going to the NICU (neonatal intensive care unit) can be a very stressful situation. It may be something you planned for, or it may be a surprise.

Know that there is a team in the hospital ready to support you, including doctors, nurses, lactation consultants, social workers, and caseworkers. There's usually a pumping room in the NICU where you can pump while you're there with your baby. There are also lactation consultants who are available to meet with you, answer your questions, and assist you with breastfeeding.

You may find it helpful to connect with other NICU moms, either in person or over social media. If you have a partner or local family and friends, consider taking shifts at the hospital so you have time to take care of yourself.

NICU tips:

- ◊ If possible, start pumping within six hours of baby's birth.
- ◊ In the first few days, hand expression can be more efficient at removing colostrum than an electric pump.
- ◊ Pump both breasts every 3 hours for 15 minutes to establish and protect your milk supply.
- ◊ Use a hospital-grade pump.

◊ Ask staff for breast milk storage guidelines and protocols for their facility.

◊ Try to do lots of skin-to-skin with baby whenever possible.

◊ Understand it may take time for baby to learn to feed at the breast.

◊ Request that a lactation consultant come see you in the NICU when you are ready to start breastfeeding.

◊ Connect with other NICU parents for community, resources, and information, both in person and online.

THE FIRST BREASTFEED

Given time, your baby could actually find your breast all on their own by army-crawling their way there from your chest. That's their natural instinct. Even if you place them on the breast yourself shortly after giving birth, you'll both benefit.

The skin-to-skin contact and suckling will trigger hormones that help your uterus contract, and there is research that finds breastfeeding within the first hour of life can lead to longer breastfeeding relationships.

You can't get a baby to breastfeed too soon, so try getting them to latch as quickly as feels comfortable. If you give birth in a hospital, you may have to advocate for yourself and insist that this happen sooner than later.

Your breasts will not feel any fuller or different than they did while you were pregnant at this point. Prior to giving birth, you may notice a clear or golden liquid coming from your breasts. (Don't worry if you don't notice it, though.) This is colostrum, and it's exactly what your newborn needs right now.

A full serving of colostrum is actually just drops—about 2 to 10 milliliters. Your baby's stomach is very small and only needs that little bit to fill up. Take a look at the stomach size comparison chart on page 73.

Newborns should nurse for a minimum of 8 to 12 times every 24 hours. From there, you'll want to time feedings from the beginning of one to the beginning of the next, aiming to breastfeed every 2 to 3 hours.

It's very important that you put baby to your breast as often as you can. The hormones your body produces every time your baby latches are what signal further milk production.

HOW TO BREAK A LATCH

Once baby has a solid latch, getting them off your nipple isn't as simple as pulling them away. In fact, that's not advisable at all.

Instead, you need to insert your finger between their gums, break the seal, and scoop your nipple out of their mouth. This is one of many reasons why it's a good idea to wash your hands before you breastfeed. You might also want to keep your nails short and polish-free.

If your baby bites down on your nipple while nursing, quickly break the latch and, with a firm tone, let baby know that hurt. Take a break from nursing. Don't smile or make it a game, or the biting might continue. For more on biting and teething, see page 160.

MOM TO MOM

"Just. Keep. Nursing. Don't feel guilty—there is nothing more important right now. If the body and the baby are riding their symbiotic relationship in harmony, it is a gift to just keep nursing."

— Erin, Troy, NY

TRACKING FEEDS

For the first few weeks, keep a daily (24-hour) log of:

- ◊ The number of breastfeeds
  - · How long the breastfeeds are
  - · Which side(s) you used
- ◊ How many bottles
  - · How many ounces in bottle
- ◊ How many wet diapers
- ◊ How many stools

There are apps available for your phone that make tracking easier and allow tracking to be shared between multiple people.

At the time of writing this book, two of the most popular breastfeeding tracking apps are Baby Feed Timer and Baby Tracker. Both are available in the Apple Store and Google Play.

Of course, the old-school way of writing stuff down in a notebook also works. If you go low-tech, one way to keep track of which breast is up next on the menu is to wear a bracelet or even a hair tie on your wrist on whatever side you last nursed. Once you latch baby to the opposite side at the next feeding, switch the bracelet over to that wrist.

DATE	TIME	SLEEP/ACTIVITY	FEEDINGS			DIAPERS	
			LEFT	RIGHT	BOTTLE	PEE	POOP

When you meet with your pediatrician or the lactation consultant, they will ask for these numbers. When you are sleep-deprived, each day starts to blur with the next one, so documenting feedings and diaper changes as they happen will make your life easier.

Many moms wonder if they should use one breast or two during each feed. The hospital will recommend you feed baby for 10 minutes on each side every time you feed. Once your milk transitions, most moms do a full feed on one side and offer the second side as "dessert." Sometimes, baby may want only one side, and sometimes baby may want both. Alternate the breast you start with to ensure that both breasts receive equal stimulation.

HOW WILL I KNOW MY BABY IS HUNGRY?

If babies could talk, parents might get a lot more sleep. Instead, we have to interpret other ways baby tries to communicate with us. There are a few clear signs baby will show when they're hungry. The sooner you can recognize and decipher these signs, the easier it will be to get into the breastfeeding flow of knowing when to feed them.

Feeding cues tend to escalate as follows:

- ◊ Opening their mouth, making sucking noises, sticking out their tongue

- ◊ Sucking on anything they can get into their mouth (their fingers, your elbow, your partner's nose)

- ◊ Rooting: rubbing their head into your chest, turning their face toward you, and opening their mouth

- ◊ Wiggling, trying to get themselves into a breast-feeding position, and moving their head from side to side

- ◊ Crying, fussing, and acting generally frustrated

Remember that these cues can signal hunger even if you just fed them (or it feels like you did). Read more about cluster feeding on page 116.

BREASTFEEDING POSITIONS

1. Start with the breastfeeding position that feels the most natural and comfortable to you.

2. Some moms like to use a breastfeeding pillow. If you're not using one you can use firm bed pillows. Either way, baby should be supported at breast level and mom should be sitting up at 90 degrees or reclining (not leaning into baby).

3. Use pillows to support your back and even a small rolled-up receiving blanket under your breasts to support them, if needed.

4. Baby should be tummy to tummy with mom.

5. Don't be afraid to switch up positions mid-feed if it's just not working for you or baby.

The cradle and cross-cradle are two common breastfeeding positions that are a great place to start when trying to figure out what feels best.

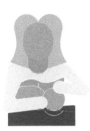

For the **CROSS-CRADLE**, one hand holds baby behind the ears, neck, and back, while the other hand sandwiches your breast. This position gives you a lot of control and allows you to help baby as they latch.

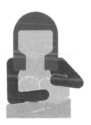

Once baby is able to sustain a deep latch, you can move to **CRADLE POSITION**. Baby rests in the crook of your arm for the cradle hold, which frees up your other hand for feeding yourself or finding something to binge-watch on Netflix.

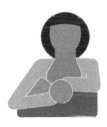

Moms with larger breasts sometimes say they prefer the **FOOTBALL HOLD**, which also happens to be a great breastfeeding position for moms recovering from a caesarean birth. It can feel easier to control your breast and see baby's latch in this position, and your baby will not rest on your tummy while nursing, but on pillows off to the side.

For the football hold, position baby along your side with their feet pointed toward your back. If they are on your right side, use your right hand behind their head to help them latch to your right breast while using your left hand to support your breast as they latch. Reverse this for the left side.

The **LAID-BACK HOLD** is very ergonomic and great to try when you have a baby who's fussy or not latching well. It can help babies feel more secure as they lie on you, tummy to tummy. This hold can also encourage babies to drop their jaws as gravity brings them to your breast and 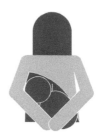 open their mouths wider as they latch. All you have to do is recline, being sure your head and shoulders are relaxed and supported, and rest baby on your tummy and chest. Use your hand to support your breast as they latch if needed, then let gravity take control.

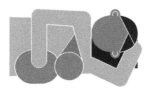 Do not be afraid of the **SIDE-LYING HOLD**. It can be a sanity and sleep saver. Place a small, firm pillow or a rolled receiving blanket behind baby's back to help keep baby from rolling away from you. Position baby on their side with their nose to your nipple, tickle their nose with your nipple, and encourage them to open wide, tilting their head back to latch.

Remember to create a safe co-sleeping space and keep any loose bedding and other pillows away from baby, even if you don't plan to fall asleep in this position.

KNOW YOUR RIGHTS AND BENEFITS!

In order to advocate for yourself and your family, you need to know your rights. There are many state and federal laws that protect families with babies and small children. Laws vary by state (so google yours), but here are key federal laws and what they mean:

PUMP AND LACTATION SUPPORT COVERAGE

Under Section 1001 of the Patient Protection and Affordable Care Act (ACA), which amends Section 2713 of the Public Health Services Act, all non-grandfathered group health plans and health insurance issuers offering group or individual coverage shall provide coverage of certain preventive services for women with no cost-sharing. This includes "comprehensive lactation support and counseling and costs of renting or purchasing breastfeeding equipment for the duration of breastfeeding,"

- ◊ **WHAT DOES THIS MEAN?** Most medical plans will provide you with a free breast pump and free lactation counseling.
- ◊ Start by calling the customer service number on your insurance card. Ask them how to get your breast pump through your insurance.

- Typically, insurance companies give you phone numbers for DME (durable medical equipment) companies. Contact them to find out what the pump options are and to place your order.
- If you'd prefer to use your breast pump benefit toward the rental of a hospital-grade pump, your insurance will often apply the same cost benefit toward the rental fees.
- Your insurance company may require you to call in your third trimester to order your pump.
- Some insurance companies will provide replacement parts for your pump, so call and ask before you buy.

◊ Ask them who you can see for lactation counseling and support (if they don't have anyone in-network, you are allowed to see a lactation consultant [IBCLC] and submit for reimbursement).

- HMO plans will often refer you to your pediatrician for lactation support.
- Some insurance providers like Kaiser and WIC may have their own resources available.
- Your pediatrician may have a lactation consultant in their office, which is covered under your insurance.

- PPO plans may have a network of lactation consultants that they are contracted with and provide you with their contact information.

PUMPING AT WORK

As of March 23, 2010, Section 4207 of the Patient Protection and Affordable Care Act (ACA), which amended Section 7 of the Fair Labor Standards Act of 1938 (29 U.S.C. 207), requires employers to provide break time and a place for most hourly wage-earning and some salaried employees (non-exempt workers) to express breast milk at work. The law states that employers must provide a "reasonable" amount of time as well as a private space other than a bath room. They are required to provide this until the employee's baby turns one year old.

◊ **WHAT DOES THIS MEAN?** Most employers must provide a locked, private pump room (not a bathroom) and appropriate time for you to pump during your work day.

FMLA

The federal Family and Medical Leave Act (FMLA) provides up to 12 weeks of unpaid, job-protected leave. There are requirements for both the employer and the employee to qualify for FMLA. Baby bonding leave under FMLA must be taken within one year of the child's birth or placement.

◊ **WHAT DOES THIS MEAN?** An employee can take up to 12 weeks of job-protected unpaid leave:

- To bond after the birth or placement of a child
- To care for a child, spouse, or parent with a serious health condition
- To deal with the employee's own serious health condition

BREASTFEEDING IN PUBLIC

All 50 states, the District of Columbia, Puerto Rico, and the Virgin Islands have laws that specifically allow women to breastfeed in any public or private location. The choice of whether or not to cover up while breastfeeding is entirely yours to make. Usually, this is influenced by how your baby handles being covered up, too. If you and baby feel more comfortable without a blanket covering your breasts and baby's head, then you are within your rights to breastfeed uncovered. On the flip side, if breastfeeding without a cover makes you uncomfortable, there is nothing wrong with using one. Breastfeed where and how you want; we just hope you're not made to feel like that should be a bathroom stall.

◊ **WHAT DOES THIS MEAN?** You can feed your baby (with or without a cover) anywhere in the United States that you are legally allowed to be!

FLEXIBLE SPENDING ACCOUNTS (FSA)

Pretax funds designated from a portion of your paycheck to cover certain types of out-of-pocket health care expenses. You can use your pretax FSA funds for:

◊ Rental or purchase of breast pumps, parts, and accessories
◊ Breastfeeding products
◊ Lactation consultations
◊ Lactation classes

BURPING, POOP, GAS, AND BARF

It's not fun dealing with a gassy baby. When gas builds up in baby and they have a hard time passing it, they can get very irritable, and this can be frustrating for the parents, too. Sometimes, gas is just a natural reaction of an immature digestive system. Other times, it can be sparked by baby swallowing air, like when they cry or when bottle-feeding. It can also be a symptom of too much milk or a forceful let-down, causing baby to gulp quickly and take in air.

There is a small possibility that gassiness correlates with a sensitivity to what mom has eaten. Remember that this is not common. Don't jump to an intense elimination diet unless you've worked with a professional to rule out other causes of gas and discomfort. Usually, food sensitivities are accompanied by excessive spit-up, diarrhea, even a cough or runny nose, and sometimes blood and mucus in their stool. Your pediatrician will be able to help you identify this.

GAS TIPS

- ◊ Growth spurts are especially gassy times. Know when they are likely to appear. Read more about growth spurts on page 113. Be aware of overfeeding during growth spurts. It will add to gas issues.

- Infant gas drops containing simethicone may help.

- Bicycling baby's legs and rocking their knees gently into each hip (alternating sides) may help.

- Try infant massage, such as the "I Love You" massage. Using two or three fingers on baby's abdomen, "draw" the letters I, an upside-down L, and an upside-down U to help draw out gas.

There are times when your baby is going to seem gassy or extra fussy and you just can't make it better. Please be sure to take care of yourself, ask for help, and check in with yourself and your partner about both of your mental health.

BURPING BABY

Generally, we don't expect breastfed babies to burp. But many moms give them a gentle burp as they switch breasts just to check, and to serve as a little "wake up" before offering the second breast. After a bottle, you probably will need to burp baby and will have an easier time doing so. Burping a bottle-fed baby is an important part of paced bottle-feeding. More on that on page 150.

HOW TO BURP:

- Hold baby so their head is aligned with your shoulder (not folded over your shoulder). Gently tap baby's back for one to two minutes. If baby needs to burp, it should come up easily. Don't worry if baby doesn't burp, especially if they don't seem to be uncomfortable.

◊ The other method is to sit baby on your lap and support them with one of your hands gently grasping their jawbone and the other hand resting on their back. You can either tap baby's back or massage baby's back in gentle circles for one to two minutes.

LET'S TALK ABOUT BARF, BABY

Babies can be super barfy. During the first three months of your baby's life, you will likely see a lot of spit-up. The lower esophageal sphincter that holds everything down in adults is not yet mature in babies, so it tends to be a two-way street. Food goes down, and it may come up. Keep in mind that spitting up for a baby is not like throwing up for an adult— it doesn't usually bother them. And spit-up often looks like more than it really is! Spit-up is the most intense during growth spurts, so be mindful not to overfeed.

When should you be concerned about spit-up?

◊ If it's affecting baby's weight gain

◊ If it's often projectile (think horror movies)

◊ If baby appears to be in pain

- If baby appears to have difficulty keeping any food down
- If the spit-up is green or yellow or has blood in it
- If baby cries for more than three hours a day or is extremely fussy
- If spit-up starts when baby is six months or older
- If baby has fewer wet diapers than usual

If you see any of these red flags, let your pediatrician know as soon as possible.

BABY POOP

You are about to become an expert on your baby's stools! Here's the scoop on baby poop.

Baby stools by age:

BLACK: Baby's first stool (meconium) is black, sticky, and tarry.

GREEN: As your breast milk starts to transition around day three to five, baby's stool will turn shades of green and appear loose.

MUSTARD: Once your breast milk has transitioned (usually by day five), baby's stools will be mustard in color and very loose. They may contain "seeds," "curds," or "strings." These poops can be small, or they might be huge blowouts that require a change of clothes. Both are super normal.

Even though these are the most common colors, it's normal to see a variety.

Stools also vary by diet:

BROWN: Formula will cause baby's stool to be shades of brown or green and to be more formed (and stinky).

VARIED: By six months, with the addition of solids, their stools will change according to what solids are moving through baby's system. They also become super stinky at this stage. (Get ready to take them straight out to the trash!)

If you're using cloth diapers, there will be a phase between the exclusively breastfed and easy-to-wash poop and the solid poop that's easy to plop into the toilet and flush. It's commonly called "peanut butter" poop because, well, you can imagine. You may want to invest in disposable diaper liners or even switch to disposables during this transition.

> When to be concerned: If you see blood or lots of mucus in baby's stool, let your pediatrician know.

You might have heard that green stools are a sign of a foremilk-hindmilk imbalance. Should you be concerned? Nope! Not if baby is happy and gaining weight appropriately.

BREASTFEEDING MULTIPLES

Breastfeeding multiples presents unique challenges. Many multiples are born premature or early term and may need time to develop feeding skills. They may spend time in the NICU and receive many bottles in the early days or weeks.

Tips for breastfeeding multiples:

◊ If babies are in the NICU, pump every 3 hours for 15 to 20 minutes to protect and establish your milk supply.

◊ Purchase a twin breastfeeding pillow.

◊ Rent a hospital-grade pump and ask your medical insurance provider to cover it.

◊ Spend time learning how to latch and feed babies individually before attempting to tandem feed.

◊ Keep them on the same schedule. When one is hungry, feed the other, too.

◊ Locate the Moms of Multiples group in your area. They are a wealth of knowledge and great support!

◊ Search for twin or multiples groups on social media.

- Ask for twin discounts! Some stores and websites will give you a discount if you are purchasing two of the same item.

- That said, keep in mind that you don't need two of everything (clothes, swings, playmats, etc.). The babies can share and rotate.

- Hire a lactation consultant to help you with latching babies and establishing supply, feeding schedules, and tandem feeding. (Remember, costs should be covered under the ACA.)

TYPES OF BREAST MILK

COLOSTRUM: For the first three to five days, you will have colostrum, which is highly concentrated, specialized breast milk full of nutrients and antibodies that are intended for your baby at this time. Colostrum is high in protein, which helps stabilize baby's blood sugar, acts as a laxative, and seals baby's GI tract so it's less permeable to infection for the rest of their life.

TRANSITIONAL MILK: Around day three to five, your milk will transition, volume will increase, and your breasts may feel fuller. For approximately two weeks, you will have transitional milk, which is a combination of colostrum and mature milk.

MATURE MILK: When baby is about three weeks old, you will have mature breast milk. The amount of breast milk you have at this point is "demand and supply." The more milk you remove from your breasts, the more you will have!

PROPER INFANT INSTALLATION

Getting a good latch is key to breastfeeding success. When baby has a good latch, feeding is comfortable for mom and baby is able to effectively transfer breast milk. Once latched, your baby's mouth should be full of breast tissue and your nipple should be touching the back of baby's palate (roof of their mouth). Baby's lips should be flanged like "fish lips" and their nose and chin should be lightly touching your breast. If the latch hurts or doesn't feel deep enough, break the latch with your finger and re-latch the baby. Don't hang out in a bad latch!

90°
×

120°
✓

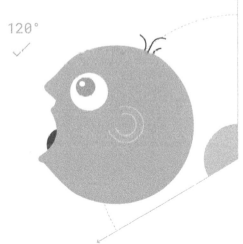

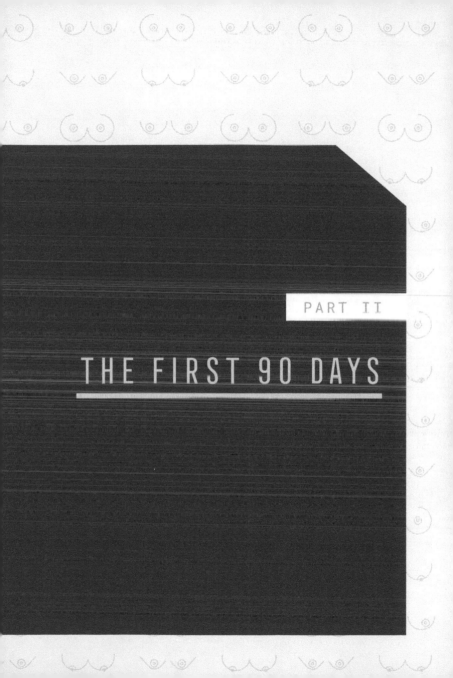

PART II

THE FIRST 90 DAYS

MENTAL HEALTH CHECK-IN

Breastfeeding doesn't just require your breasts. Your whole body and mind are activated for this task. It's important that you're not only taking care of your nipples and your milk supply but also checking in with the rest of you.

We already touched on "baby blues." The term is used to describe common feelings of sadness that come on as your hormones fluctuate and life adjusts after baby's arrival. The baby blues may make your cry for two to three weeks after giving birth, but they won't make you cry all day for weeks on end, for example.

If you find that you're feeling sad, anxious, angry, or mentally off in any other way for more than a couple of weeks, you may be dealing with a postpartum mood disorder that needs treatment.

Postpartum mood disorders, like postpartum depression, postpartum anxiety, and postpartum OCD, can affect as many as one in seven mothers. Research suggests this number is even higher for women of color.

You, your partner, and other supportive people in your life should look for the following symptoms:

◊ Feeling overwhelmed or hopeless
◊ Feeling sad or empty
◊ Guilt

- ◊ Panic
- ◊ Racing thoughts
- ◊ Inability to relax
- ◊ Sleeping a lot or not much at all
- ◊ Loss of appetite
- ◊ Loss of focus
- ◊ Rage
- ◊ Fear
- ◊ Disturbing thoughts you can't shake
- ◊ Intense desire to keep checking on baby or other things
- ◊ Unprovoked inability to trust those around you

Even if you're not experiencing any symptoms of these mood disorders before or at your six-week postpartum checkup—the time when most providers will ask you about them—they can still set in up to a year after your baby is born (especially when you experience hormonal shifts like when you wean from breastfeeding and/or menstruation returns).

Society seems to talk most about postpartum depression, but new research is showing that postpartum anxiety may be just as common or even more prevalent than postpartum depression. Don't chalk up rage and worry to being an exhausted and concerned new parent if those symptoms are interfering with your life.

PMADs (perinatal mood and anxiety disorders) also affect dads, partners, same-sex couples, and adoptive parents. Often, the partner's symptoms are delayed as the initial time and attention is focused on the mother and baby. Risk factors are biological (genetics and family mental health history), psychological (trauma, previous depression, and anxiety), and social (relationships, support, finances, or stress level). The bottom line is that PMADs can affect anyone.

If you recognize that you or your partner are dealing with any of the above symptoms at any time, get in touch with your health care provider. You can reach out to your OB-GYN, midwife, or family physician. Be honest and upfront about what you're feeling, and know that these are symptoms of a treatable illness. This is not a reflection of your worth or capability as a parent.

There are breastfeeding-safe medications that can help treat all these mood disorders. Two that are commonly prescribed for breastfeeding moms are Zoloft and Lexapro. Be sure to discuss any medication you're considering with your doctor.

If you don't have a medical provider you can talk to about these symptoms, please reach out to Postpartum Support International.

Phone: (800) 944-4773
Text: (503) 894-9453
Or visit Postpartum.net.

INSTALLING AND OPTIMIZING A BREAST PUMP

If there are no complications with breastfeeding in the first few weeks, the ideal time to introduce pumping and bottle-feeding is between four and six weeks. However, some moms may need to start pumping earlier if:

- Baby is in NICU
- Mom and baby are separated
- Baby needs to be supplemented
- Mom's milk has not transitioned
- Mom has very sore or damaged nipples
- Mom is working on increasing supply
- Mom has multiples

Moms often worry that early introduction of bottles will ruin breastfeeding. Using the paced bottle-feeding technique and giving appropriate amounts in the bottle will help ensure that baby is able to go back and forth between breast and bottle. For more information on the paced bottle-feeding technique, visit https://kellymom.com/bf/pumpingmoms /feeding-tools/bottle-feeding/.

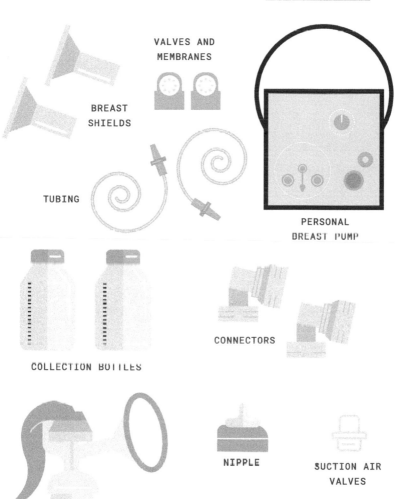

VALVES AND
MEMBRANES

BREAST
SHIELDS

TUBING

PERSONAL
BREAST PUMP

COLLECTION BOTTLES

CONNECTORS

MANUAL BREAST PUMP

NIPPLE

SUCTION AIR
VALVES

SEALING DISK

DUST COVER

TEAM LIFT!

Breastfeeding can feel isolating when, in fact, it should be a team effort. The best way to set yourself up for long-term success is to build a strong support network before baby is born. When you're pregnant, make sure your medical team knows you intend to breastfeed. If you deliver in a hospital, request a visit from the lactation consultant on staff as early as possible. You can follow this up with in-home or in-office lactation consultant visits or arrange for this if you have a home birth. This is often covered by your insurance thanks to the Affordable Care Act. Your partner may not be the one with the lactating breasts, but they can still help by making sure you have water and plenty of food you can eat with one hand. Finally, the emotional support of people around you can go very far. Let your loved ones know how much breastfeeding means to you and ask them to encourage you whenever they can.

AFTERMARKET ACCESSORIES

BREAST PUMPS: Breast pumps are devices that extract milk from lactating breasts. There are four types of pumps: hospital-grade, personal, manual, and silicone bulb.

HOSPITAL-GRADE PUMPS: Recommended for moms who are separated from their baby or have multiples, very damaged nipples, or low milk supply. These are multiuser pumps and are usually rentals.

PERSONAL PUMPS: Recommended for most moms who are pumping at work or for daily bottles. These may be "open system" (meant for a single user) or "closed system" (safe for multiusers).

MANUAL PUMP: Recommended for occasional or emergency use.

SILICONE "BULB" PUMPS: Recommended for easy collection of breast milk while breastfeeding the baby. The Haakaa is an example of this kind of pump. Some moms also use it as a collection device to hand-express into.

HANDS-FREE PUMPING BRA: Holds collection bottles in place at mom's breasts so mom's hands can be free to multitask.

NURSING PADS: Absorb milk from leaking breasts. Typically only worn in the first six weeks. They come in cloth, bamboo, and disposable versions.

NIPPLE SHIELDS: Thin, silicone covers that go over the nipple while baby breastfeeds. They can help with flat or sore/damaged nipples, assisting with baby's latch, and transitioning a bottle-preferring baby back to breast. They should always be used under the guidance of a lactation consultant.

NIPPLE SHELLS: Keep bra/shirt off sore and damaged nipples.

NIPPLE CREAM AND LANOLIN: Used to help prevent and heal sore nipples.

BREASTFEEDING PILLOW: Helps create a stable "table" to position baby when latching and breastfeeding.

NURSING COVER: Gives mom privacy when breastfeeding.

NURSING BRA/SHIRTS/CLOTHES: Allow easy access for baby to breastfeed.

BREAST MILK STORAGE BAGS: Used to store breast milk in the freezer.

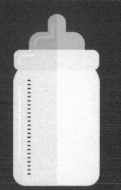

LANOLIN

MILK STORAGE BAGS

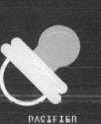

BOTTLE

PACIFIER

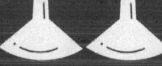

NIPPLE SHIELDS

PERSONAL
BREAST PUMP

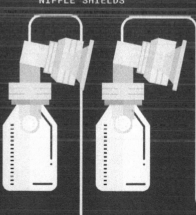

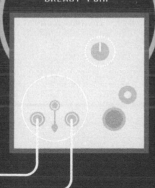

BABIES LOSE WEIGHT AFTER BIRTH! IT'S OK!

Once home, mom and baby will fall into a breastfeeding rhythm. Moms typically have the most milk in the early morning and less later in the day or evening. In the first six weeks, it's very common for baby to feed frequently at night. Around six to eight weeks, babies will generally start sleeping a little longer at night and squeeze in more feeds during the day. Babies should always feed a minimum of eight times every 24 hours, but once they are back to their birth weight, getting at least four to six wet diapers each day, and gaining weight appropriately, you no longer have to wake baby up. Instead, follow their lead.

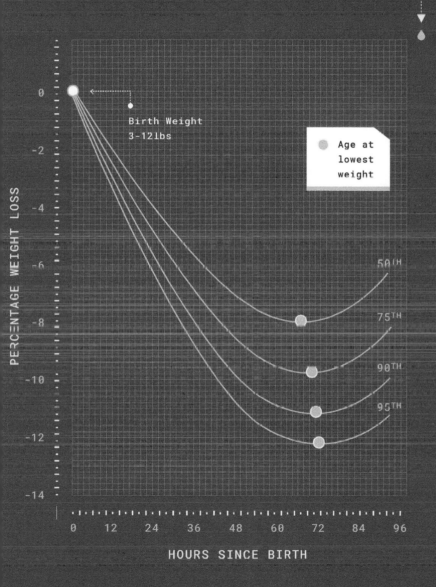

Birth Weight
3-12lbs

Age at
lowest
weight

50TH

75TH

90TH

95TH

PERCENTAGE WEIGHT LOSS

0

-2

-4

-6

-8

-10

-12

-14

0   12   24   36   48   60   72   84   96

HOURS SINCE BIRTH

CO-SLEEPING WITH A BREASTFED BABY

Co-sleeping is a personal and family decision, and you should do your research before you consider it. It can be convenient and comfortable, but it's not without risks.

The American Academy of Pediatrics says the safest place for a baby to sleep is on their back on a firm surface with no loose bedding or pillows. This is typically in a crib or bassinet in their parent's bedroom for at least the first six months. The AAP also recognizes that many breastfeeding parents end up co-sleeping at some point.

If you think you may fall asleep while breastfeeding, the recommended location to do so is actually your bed, but keep safe co-sleeping practices in mind. Just like a safe crib, the bed you co-sleep in should have a firm mattress and no covers, sheets, or pillows that can come in contact with the baby. Adults in the bed should not use drugs or alcohol while co-sleeping, and other children or pets should not share the bed.

If you can safely and comfortably create a co-sleeping routine that works for your family, it can make breastfeeding more enjoyable, especially through the night.

YOUR MILK SUPPLY

Moms often worry that they won't have enough milk. Good news: 90 percent of first-time moms have enough milk to feed their babies! If baby is feeding 8 to 12 times a day for approximately 20 to 25 minutes, has at least four to six wet diapers, and is gaining weight appropriately, that means you have enough milk and you guys are doing great.

Signs of a good breastfeed:

- ◊ You observe baby actively sucking and swallowing.
- ◊ You may hear audible swallows.
- ◊ Your breasts feel softer after a feed.
- ◊ Baby seems satiated after the feed.

If you are worried you don't have enough milk, contact a lactation consultant. They will evaluate your anatomy, baby's anatomy, your latch, your feeding history, your medical history, and your supply. They may recommend herbs, a feeding and pumping plan, or another intervention to increase your supply.

GENERATING QUALITY FUEL

Although studies show moms need an additional 300 to 500 calories per day while breastfeeding (compared to a pre-pregnancy diet), most moms accomplish this by eating to satiety and maintaining three meals plus a couple of snacks each day. There should be no need to count calories. There is no specific diet you need to maintain while breastfeeding, and there's no list of foods you can't eat (advice to not eat spicy or gassy foods is based on myths). If you're having a hard time getting in enough calories:

- Try to focus on eating calorie-dense foods like nuts, cheese, avocado, butter, and sauces.

- Try to increase the number of snacks you eat during the day by keeping easy, ready-to-eat foods nearby while you breastfeed.

- Ask friends and family to bring pre-prepared food (bonus if there's extra to go in the freezer for later).

- Try overnight oats for breakfast. They are easy to make in advance and may even boost your milk supply.

Similarly, adequate hydration can usually be accomplished by drinking enough water to satisfy thirst. However, most moms find they are very thirsty while breastfeeding or pumping, so keep a full water bottle nearby!

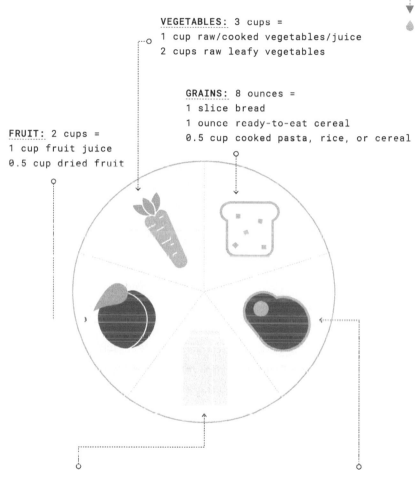

VEGETABLES: 3 cups =
1 cup raw/cooked vegetables/juice
2 cups raw leafy vegetables

GRAINS: 8 ounces =
1 slice bread
1 ounce ready-to-eat cereal
0.5 cup cooked pasta, rice, or cereal

FRUIT: 2 cups =
1 cup fruit juice
0.5 cup dried fruit

DAIRY: 3 cups =
1 cup milk
8 ounces yogurt
1.5 onces cheese
2 ounces processed cheese

MEAT AND BEANS: 6.5 ounces =
1 ounce lean meat, poultry, or fish
0.25 cup cooked dry beans
0.5 ounce nuts / 1 egg
1 tablespoon peanut butter

DEALING WITH DISCOMFORT AND PAIN

It is normal to feel a little nipple discomfort in the couple of weeks when baby first latches. Typically, any slight pain or discomfort subsides within a few seconds. Latching should feel better and better each day. If you want to cry, if you're dreading breastfeeding, or if your nipples are cracked and bleeding, it's time to get help! Common reasons for sore nipples include shallow latch, mom's and/or baby's position, long breastfeeds, and tongue-tie.

A full breastfeed should last approximately 20 to 25 minutes. Once baby is taking long pauses (five seconds or more) between bursts of sucking, they are in the comfort (non-nutritive) stage. If you have sore nipples, you should minimize comfort sucking, breaking the latch when baby gets to that point. If baby is taking a bottle, try folding in a few pumping and bottle-feeding sessions in place of a breastfeed, which will give your nipples a break.

Some moms report that lanolin and nipple creams help their nipples heal faster. (Pro tip: Studies show breast milk is even better than nipple creams and lanolin—and it's free!)

A lactation consultant can help you triage sore nipples and make a plan for more comfortable breastfeeding. This cost should be covered under the Affordable Care Act. If your insurance doesn't cover it, ask the lactation consultant if they will give you a cash discount. Breastfeeding support groups are available at most hospitals and are usually free or low-cost.

Another source of discomfort in the early days is uterine contractions when you breastfeed. This is an important health benefit, as the uterus contracting helps prevent postpartum hemorrhage. Breastfeeding helps that process happen faster. These contractions will likely increase in intensity after each birth. If you are concerned about the amount of postpartum bleeding you're experiencing, contact your OB-GYN or midwife.

COMMON PROBLEMS AND SOLUTIONS

THRUSH: A fungal infection that both mom and baby can get. The three places it appears are on mom's nipples, inside of baby's cheeks and tongue, and on baby's bottom as a diaper rash. When mom has thrush on her nipples, it usually burns and feels very itchy. You usually see flaky skin around the nipple and areola. On baby, it can appear as thick patches on the tongue and on the inside of their cheeks that won't wipe off easily. Most of the time, thrush needs to be treated with an antifungal prescription. And it is most effective when mom and baby are treated simultaneously. More information in CODE 028 (page 156).

PLUGGED DUCTS: A plugged duct is when breast milk gets stuck in a milk duct. If it isn't cleared within 24 to 48 hours, it can turn into mastitis. This affects mom only, can cause supply to dip on the affected side, and is very painful. The main treatment for a plugged duct is to physically break up the plug and clear it from the duct. More information in CODE 023 (page 142).

MASTITIS: Mastitis is a breast infection. Symptoms include fever of 101.3°F or greater, chills, body aches, redness, swelling, and tenderness in breast. Most often, it's caused by a plugged duct that mom was not able to clear. If mom cannot clear the plug within 24 hours of onset of fever, she needs to see her doctor for antibiotics. More information in CODE 023 (page 142).

CRACKED NIPPLES: Cracked, damaged nipples are often the result of a bad or shallow latch, long breastfeeds, a baby who is teething, distracted baby, tongue-tie, or a pumping issue. If the damage is severe and not healing within a couple of days using home healing measures, mom should schedule an appointment with a lactation consultant for help. For more information check out CODE 024 (page 146).

DO NOT PANIC IF YOUR BREASTS DO THIS

Here are some things your lactating breasts might do that may catch you off guard.

They may grow so large and get so hard that they resemble melons three to five days after your baby is born when your milk transitions. It's normal to find this (A) hilarious, (B) horrifying, and (C) painful. For C, refer to page 103 for tips on how to relieve engorgement.

They may spontaneously let-down anytime you hear not only your baby cry but any baby cry. That strange newborn in aisle five who just let out a wail may be the reason for the two wet spots on your shirt at checkout.

Your breasts don't turn off just because you've switched from feeding a baby to feeling sexy. In fact, the hormone released during orgasm is the same one that signals your body to let-down. In other words, you might want to warn your partner about your new spray features before climax.

Most moms report that their supply increases right after sex—a nice benefit!

Another consideration regarding sex while breastfeeding is what most moms refer to as being "touched out." It's well within the range of normal to cringe at the thought of your partner touching your breasts (or any other part of you) after you've had a baby suctioned to your nipples half the day.

MOM TO MOM

"Don't assume that each kid will be the same. I had very different breastfeeding journeys with each kid."

— Elisa, Los Alamos, NM

BABY FEVER WHILE BREASTFEEDING?!

Just because you're breastfeeding exclusively doesn't mean you can't get pregnant, even if your period hasn't made a postpartum appearance yet. It's not common, but a small percentage of women get pregnant during their first postpartum ovulation.

BIRTH CONTROL AND TRYING TO CONCEIVE WHILE BREASTFEEDING

If you're hoping to avoid another pregnancy while breastfeeding, you can only rely on exclusive breastfeeding as a form of birth control with a 98 to 99.5 percent effective rate if your baby is younger than six months old, your period has not returned, and your baby is exclusively breastfed (at your breast, no bottles) on cue throughout the day and night. The efficacy of breastfeeding as birth control decreases as each of those factors change, even just a little bit.

Make sure your OB-GYN knows you're breastfeeding if you're going on birth control pills. In general, breastfeeding moms want to avoid pills containing estrogen, which can lower your supply. Progesterone-only pills can as well, although it's not as common. Keep an eye on your supply when you start birth control!

Abrupt changes in your breastfeeding schedule, like a baby sleeping through the night or suddenly skipping an afternoon feed because they are eating solid foods, can signal to your body that it's time to bring your period back.

After your period returns, it may still take a few months for your fertility to return, meaning these may be periods that are not accompanied by ovulation. With time, your cycles should return to normal pre-pregnancy fertility. It is usually not necessary to wean in order to conceive again.

PREGNANCY WHILE BREASTFEEDING

If you do become pregnant while you're breastfeeding, it's very likely you can safely continue breastfeeding if you're comfortable doing so. In some rare cases, like a high-risk pregnancy, your OB-GYN or midwife may advise you to stop breastfeeding, but it's generally considered safe to do while pregnant.

A common challenge is balancing the physical side effects of pregnancy with breastfeeding. Your nipples and breasts will become more tender, and nausea may increase with let-down. This is a great opportunity to master side-lying nursing so you can rest and breastfeed at the same time.

You should be able to consume enough calories to sustain a healthy pregnancy, produce breast milk, and nourish yourself simply by listening to your hunger cues and eating to satiety. Be sure to stay hydrated, too.

If you tandem feed after baby is born, meaning you are breastfeeding both your older child and the new baby, you may need to increase your caloric intake to maintain your milk supply. Again, listen to your body and eat if you're hungry. Fatigue can be a sign you're not getting enough calories. (It can also be a sign that you have a newborn. Either way, treat yourself.)

Your milk supply will likely dip early to midway through your pregnancy, and your milk will transition from mature milk to colostrum in the second half of pregnancy. Around this time, your older baby may decide they don't like the taste of your milk. Toddlers may even tell you it's yucky. Not all babies and toddlers self-wean at this stage, but some do.

The golden liquid known as colostrum that is so important for newborn babies (more on page 39) will be back in full force in time for your next baby, and as with the last baby, it will transition to mature milk over the next week.

MOM TO MOM

"It doesn't have to be all or nothing! Both of my babies ended up getting bottles at one time or another because of struggles with latching. Some of those bottles have been bottles of formula because I had trouble pumping enough to keep up. With my first I eventually stopped nursing because I couldn't build a backup stash. It still breaks my heart to think about; I could have kept going happily combo feeding. I'm so glad my 15-week-old is getting the best of both worlds—all the benefits of my milk, plus I'm confident that she's getting enough and less stressed over pumping."

— Autumn, Columbus, OH

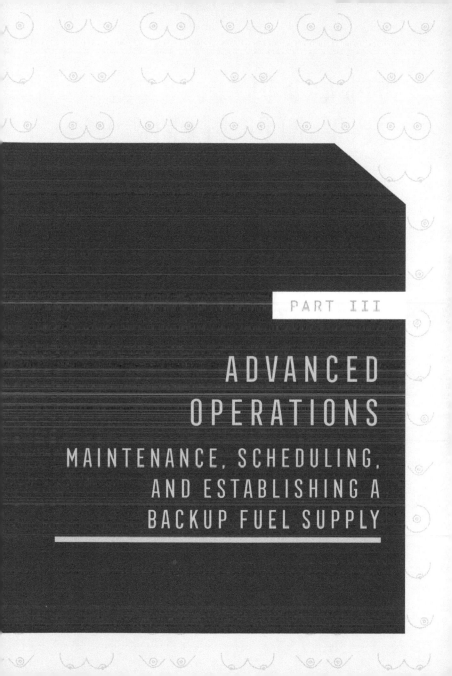

ADVANCED OPERATIONS

MAINTENANCE, SCHEDULING, AND ESTABLISHING A BACKUP FUEL SUPPLY

DEMAND FEEDING VS. SCHEDULED FEEDINGS

When mom and baby are together and most feeds are at the breast, you'll want to follow baby's schedule. Watch for feeding cues, and feed on demand. (More on feeding and hunger cues on page 23.) Most moms have more milk in the morning, so babies will do big feeds in the morning and smaller feeds as the day progresses. Cluster feeding in the late afternoon or evening is completely normal. Babies are usually "tanking up" for the night. Encouraging cluster feeding will usually equal better sleep for everyone at night! This is also referred to as the "witching hour" but it's more like two to four hours. If you observe your baby's feeding pattern you will see their schedule emerge. They tend to feed around the same time of day if you follow their lead. (Refer to page 116 for more information on cluster feeding.)

If mom returns to work outside the home, baby will usually get more bottle feeds. If mom is away for an eight-hour day, baby will typically need a three-ounce bottle every three hours while separated from mom. And mom will pump both breasts every three hours for 15 minutes while apart. Generally, mom and baby breastfeed when they are back together in the evening and in the morning.

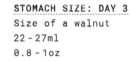

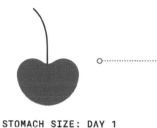

STOMACH SIZE: DAY 1
Size of a cherry
5 - 7ml
0.1 - 0.2oz

STOMACH SIZE: DAY 3
Size of a walnut
22 - 27ml
0.8 - 1oz

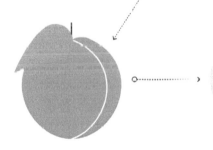

STOMACH SIZE: DAY 7
Size of an apricot
45 - 60ml
1.5 - 2oz

STOMACH SIZE: DAY 30
Size of an egg
80 - 150ml
2.5 - 5oz

ESTABLISHING AND MAINTAINING A BACKUP FOOD SUPPLY

Most moms want baby to be able to take the breast and a bottle. If you'd like to begin pumping and bottle-feeding, the best time to get started is when baby is approximately four to six weeks old. By four weeks, breastfeeding is considered firmly established. If you wait much longer than six weeks, baby may decide they don't want a bottle. You definitely don't want to wait until right before you return to the office!

Start pumping two to three days before you plan to give your first bottle. Pump for 10 minutes immediately following a morning breastfeed (you have the most milk in the morning) and put that milk in the refrigerator. After two to three days you should have enough for a couple of bottles. Now, you can start pumping once a day for your daily bottle. When your baby starts taking a bottle, you can either pump in place of the breastfeed or pump after any breastfeed and skip the pump session when baby gets the bottle.

Using the Haakaa or a similar silicone suction manual pump is another way you can start collecting milk. Silicone pumps attach to your other breast while you are breast-feeding. It doesn't take any extra time, and it's an easy way to start building your stash.

It's a good idea to own a quality personal breast pump. (Pro tip: Your medical insurance company should provide one for you under the Affordable Care Act.) That's the pump you'll use most of the time at home, and at work if you're returning to your job.

The manual pump is also your "emergency pump" to throw in a bag when you leave the house or use on an airplane, in a car, or anywhere you might not be able to use your personal breast pump. Don't leave home without it!

STORING BREAST MILK

A breast milk storage shortcut that is often shared is the 5-5-5 rule. Breast milk is good for five hours at room temperature, five days in the fridge, and five months in the freezer. The real numbers are a little different but you won't go wrong with this rule, and it's easy to remember.

If you're ever unsure whether breast milk is still good, the "sniff test" is a reliable way to find out. Breast milk will smell sour and rancid if it's bad. You can also move milk "forward." For example, if it's been in the refrigerator for four days and you're not sure you'll get to it, move it to the freezer.

Other guidelines:

- ◊ Breast milk should be the same temperature when you combine it.
- ◊ Never add fresh or refrigerated breast milk to frozen breast milk.
- ◊ Never refreeze breast milk.
- ◊ Thawed breast milk is good for 24 hours.
- ◊ If your thawed breast milk contains even one ice crystal, it's still considered frozen. This is super important in cases of power outages or if the freezer door gets left open.
- ◊ If your thawed breast milk smells soapy or metallic, contact a lactation consultant.

Common supplies used for storing breast milk:

- ◊ Breast milk storage bags (for freezer)
- ◊ Dry erase marker to date storage containers in refrigerator
- ◊ Insulated, zippered lunch bag and two frozen packs (for transporting milk)

There are several breast milk storage systems on the market that will help with storing and organizing your frozen bags of milk. One great hack is a low-cost solution:

Get a small to medium gift bag. It should fit in your freezer with enough room for you to reach in and drop a breast milk bag at the top.

On one of the narrow sides at the bottom of the bag, cut a hole just big enough for a full, frozen bag of milk to come out of. After you seal and mark the date on your breast milk bag with an indelible marker, drop it into the bag so it lies flat. If you retrieve bags of milk from the hole at the bottom of the bag, you'll always be grabbing the oldest bag first. This storage method also keeps your bags of milk flat as they freeze, preventing them from turning into frozen rocks of breast milk.

DEFROSTING FROZEN BREAST MILK

A bag of frozen breast milk can take about 12 hours to thaw in the refrigerator.

◊ You can also thaw the bag of breast milk by holding it under warm (not hot), running water.

◊ Never let breast milk thaw at room temperature.

◊ Never use a microwave or boiling water to thaw frozen breast milk. Not only do you risk scalding yourself or baby if it gets too hot, heat can also damage the nutritional properties of breast milk.

◊ Once the breast milk has thawed, it should immediately be put in the refrigerator for up to 24 hours, fed to baby within two hours, or discarded.

BREASTFEEDING, ALCOHOL, AND SMOKING?

Alcohol

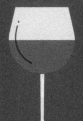

Current research shows occasional use of alcohol (one or two drinks) does not appear to be harmful to a breastfeeding baby. Generally, the rule of thumb is if you are sober enough to drive, you are sober enough to breastfeed. Alcohol does not build up in the breast milk or need to be pumped out prior to feeding baby. The milk alcohol levels decrease as your blood alcohol level decreases. So when you feel sober, it's okay to feed the baby.

If you are away from baby and drinking, you will still need to pump on a regular schedule to protect your milk supply. (Pro tip: Since there's alcohol in that milk, it wouldn't be safe for baby to ingest, but some moms save it to add to baby's next bath. Breast milk is great for the skin!)

The greater risk when it comes to alcohol consumption is making sure you are not impaired and endangering baby.

Smoking

All mothers are encouraged to quit smoking. The more a mother smokes, the greater the health risks are for her and her baby.

Babies who live with adults who smoke are seven times more likely to die from SIDS (sudden infant death syndrome). They may also experience ear infections, croup, asthma, and pneumonia more than babies who do not live with adults who smoke.

But a breastfeeding mother who finds herself unable or unwilling to quit should still breastfeed her baby. In fact, breastfeeding can actually decrease the negative effects of exposure to smoke on their lungs.

Smoking mothers should:

◊ Cut down or quit, if possible
◊ Smoke right after a breastfeed (avoid smoking right before or during)
◊ Smoke outside and away from baby, if possible
◊ Change clothes after smoking (shower if possible)

EXTRACTION AND STORAGE ON THE JOB

Approximately four to six weeks before your back-to-work date, you should start storing a little extra milk in the freezer. Twenty to 30 ounces is a great target amount for a stash. The purpose of this stash is to give you a little wiggle room when you return to work. Most moms accomplish this by doing an extra pump (usually in the morning) right after a breastfeed and sending that milk straight to the freezer.

Once mom returns to work, baby will typically get more bottles during the day. If mom is working an eight-hour day, baby will typically need a 3-ounce bottle every three hours while separated from mom. Mom will pump both breasts every three hours for 15 minutes while apart. Generally, mom and baby breastfeed when they are back together in the evening and in the morning.

Tips for pumping at work:

- ◊ Speak to human resources before you return to make sure there's a pumping room available for you.

- ◊ It's normal to experience a small dip in your supply for the first couple of weeks after returning to work.

- ◊ If you work in an office with calendared meetings, put your pump breaks on the schedule.

◊ Coordinate pump breaks with other pumping coworkers.

◊ A hands-free pumping bra can free you up to eat or continue working while you pump.

◊ Hand massaging your breasts before and during pumping ("hands-on pumping") can dramatically increase pumped volumes.

◊ If you find it difficult to let-down while you're away from baby, call the caregiver to check in, or look at videos or pictures of your baby.

Caregiver tips:

◊ Make sure the caregiver is bottle-feeding the same way you bottle-feed (same technique, same length of time, same breaks).

◊ Watch the amount fed while you're away. The average should be around 1 ounce for every hour you're gone.

◊ Share breast milk storage guidelines with the caregiver so they follow the same rules you would.

*** Federal and state laws protect your right to take pump breaks and pump at work. Know your rights! (Visit page 27 for an extensive list of your rights.)

TRAVELING FOR BUSINESS

TSA guidelines state that reasonable amounts of both breast milk and formula do not count toward your liquid allowance when you carry them on the plane. Additionally, your pump does not count as a carry-on, as it's a medical device. That said, TSA at every airport varies, and some are better at handling breast milk and breast pumps than others. It doesn't hurt to let the TSA agents at the bag-screening area know you are sending through a breast pump and/or bags of breast milk.

It's also always a good idea to bring a manual pump when traveling by plane, just in case you don't have access to electricity. You may even want to pack a scarf or muslin blanket in your bag so you can pump in your seat if you're comfortable doing so.

If you've been exclusively breastfeeding your baby, you'll need to pump both breasts every three hours for 15 minutes. Most moms can go a little longer at night. Bring your lactation consultant's phone number with you in case you get a plugged duct or run into any other complications while traveling.

Moms who travel for work can bring their pumped milk back with them. Packing breast milk in a cooler with dry ice works well for the return trip home. In a pinch, fill your cooler with ice from the food court once you're past security.

There are also services for hire that will ship your breast milk back for you. Ask your human resources department if that's a benefit your company provides.

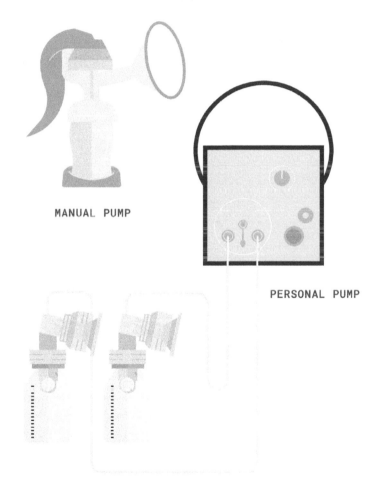

MANUAL PUMP

PERSONAL PUMP

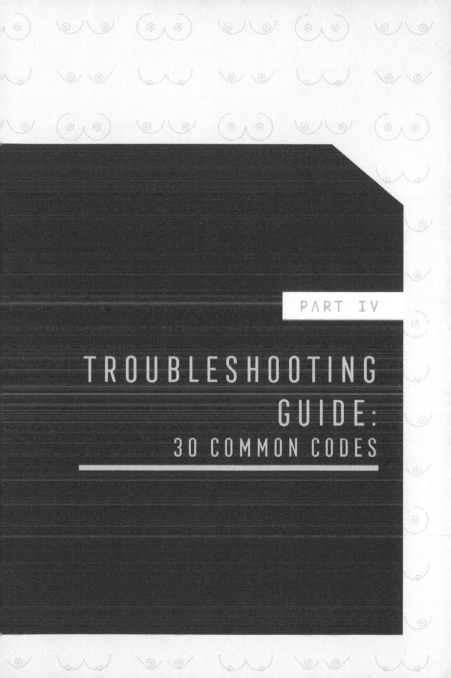

PART IV

TROUBLESHOOTING
GUIDE:
30 COMMON CODES

I NEED SOMEONE TO HELP ME WITH BREASTFEEDING!

DIAGNOSTICS: Any difficulties with breastfeeding, concerns that breastfeeding isn't going well

Breastfeeding is natural, but it doesn't come naturally for many of us. Most moms need a support network— a village—while breastfeeding. They need other people to show them how to do it. They need people in their life who are supportive of it and who will cheer them on when they need an extra push. And they need medical professionals, like lactation consultants, who can help them navigate trials and challenges.

It's great if you can begin to piece together this network before you give birth. Be sure you get a visit from the on-staff lactation consultant at the hospital before you leave and inquire about drop-in times or support groups for when you're home. Get recommendations for a good on-call, emergency lactation consultant or look up online lactation consultant services you can use. This is a good time to research what, if any, lactation services your medical insurance covers. If no services are covered, try to set aside

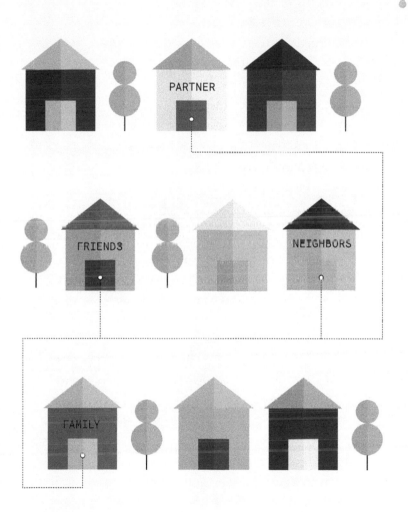

CODE 001:

PARTNER

FRIENDS

NEIGHBORS

FAMILY

enough funds to pay for one or two emergency lactation consultations before baby is born.

Breastfeeding support groups are a great place not only to get help with breastfeeding but also to meet other parents with babies around the same age as yours. Making friends with people in the same situation as you can help you get through breastfeeding challenges, and these can become real, long-term friendships. Your kids will be having playdates in the blink of an eye.

TROUBLESHOOTING TIPS

There are several layers of breastfeeding support available in most communities!

- ◊ Lactation consultants can be found in private practice, hospitals, and pediatrician offices. International Board Certified Lactation Consultants (IBCLCs) are the gold standard in lactation professionals, and they are well trained to assess breastfeeding difficulties and develop a plan of care. This "Find a Lactation Consultant" directory is current and easy to use: www.ilca. org. (Fun fact: Lactation consultants who are IBCLCs should be covered under your insurance. Call the customer service number on your insurance card and ask how your provider fulfills the federal mandate to cover lactation support under the Affordable Care Act.)

The National Women's Law Center has a great tool kit on your lactation coverage under the ACA called "Getting the Coverage You Deserve."

◊ Breastfeeding support groups are usually free or low cost. They are typically run by lactation consultants. In addition to having access to breastfeeding advice, you'll meet other local breastfeeding moms and have the chance to build a support network.

◊ Doulas and lactation educators are often able to help triage basic latch and positioning issues and provide breastfeeding information and education.

◊ La Leche League offers free peer-to-peer support provided by volunteers. Many of them meet once a month In parks and churches. This Is another great opportunity to find your breastfeeding community and receive breastfeeding help and support.

◊ Help is out there!

I'M EXHAUSTED!

__DIAGNOSTICS__: Newborn baby in the house

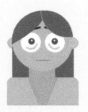 Sleep deprivation is no joke when you have a newborn. When that newborn is relying on your body to feed them, your exhaustion can compound. Remember, your most important job right now is feeding, taking care of, and getting to know your baby. Dishes, laundry, errands, even washing your hair can all take several seats.

Instead of feeling worthless or like you're getting nothing done, reframe this time as one of productivity that requires you to sit still. Your body is, in fact, doing a ton of work even when you hold a baby all day and catch up on the latest season of *Queer Eye*.

TROUBLESHOOTING TIPS

- ◊ Try to nap. Some moms find it more restful to nap near or with their baby.

- ◊ Often, the nights are harder, so lie low during the day.

- Tag-team with your partner or support person.

- Focus on taking little moments of self-care where you can (cup of tea, breath of fresh air, favorite snack, call with a friend).

- Know the timing of growth spurts and developmental leaps (check out the Wonder Weeks app). These will be difficult weeks, but it'll help if you can make a plan for when they come.

- Outsource whatever you can. For example, use grocery delivery services.

- Keep a "fridge list" of to-dos so that when friends and family call and ask how they can help, you're ready!

- Consider asking a friend to coordinate a "meal train" for when you come home.

- Remember that one serving of caffeine a day is compatible with breastfeeding, if that's your thing.

Exhaustion will pass eventually (or ease up, leaving you simply tired). We're not telling you to "savor every moment" because this phase is hard and it's okay to not enjoy it all the time. That said, know that this is a phase; you will have fond memories of holding your newborn but you won't look back and care if you did the dishes or not.

WILL MY CAESAREAN DELIVERY RUIN BREASTFEEDING?

DIAGNOSTICS: Baby's size or position, mom or baby medical issue

A caesarean delivery is major abdominal surgery! It takes longer to recover from a C-section than a vaginal delivery. In addition to adjusting to your new life with a newborn, you're going to need to learn how to do those things while recovering from surgery. Although recovery commonly takes weeks, you should feel a little better each day. You will soon discover that your abdomen is involved in everything from laughing to rolling over. Get help for yourself and for baby. Make sure you ask for a hand when getting up and sitting down. Take it slow, and don't push yourself too hard.

TROUBLESHOOTING TIPS

◊ If baby is delivered via C-section, you may be separated from them for a few hours immediately following the birth. That's OK! Breastfeed as soon as you are back together.

- Between feeds, keep baby skin-to-skin on your chest. This is the most comfortable place for baby and helps regulate their temperature. You'll also be sensitive to baby's feeding cues.

- Baby will often start "bobbing" their head, looking for the breast when they're ready to feed.

- You may find that your breast milk transitions a little later than with a vaginal delivery.

- You'll probably find that the football hold is the most comfortable because it gets baby off your abdominal area, which might be tender following surgery.

- Side-lying is another good position.

- Ask the nurse or lactation consultant to come in (each time if needed) and help position baby and assist with latch.

- The medications your doctor prescribes for you will be compatible with breastfeeding. In fact, being in pain can inhibit your let-down, so take what you need!

- When you get home, keep in mind that you are recovering from abdominal surgery. Get extra help as needed.

IT HURTS WHEN MY BABY LATCHES!

DIAGNOSTICS: Shallow latch, breastfeeding position, long breastfeeds, flat or inverted nipples, tongue-tie

There's a myth that breastfeeding pain is normal and it's just something you have to get through. We're here to tell you not to believe that.

Of course, when your nipples aren't used to being sucked on multiple times a day, they will have to adjust, and that can cause some discomfort and even mild pain for a short time. This shouldn't interfere with your breastfeeding relationship, though.

The majority of long-lasting pain while breastfeeding is caused by an improper latch. There are many reasons a baby may not master their latch. This part—trying to figure out what's keeping them from latching on right—can be frustrating, but with some patience and, possibly, some help from a lactation consultant, you can pinpoint the issue and work to correct it quickly.

TROUBLESHOOTING TIPS

◊ Before latching baby, compress your breast tissue ("sandwich") with the hand closest to your breast.

◊ Position baby tummy to tummy with you, so their nose is aligned with your nipple.

◊ With your other hand, hold baby firmly behind the ears, neck, and back.

◊ Run your nipple over baby's mouth and nose until they open wide.

◊ Wait for a big, wide-open mouth, and then bring baby to your breast with their bottom lip connecting first, followed by the top lip. This allows you to fold your breast into baby's mouth.

◊ Your nipple should land at the back of baby's hard palate, and their mouth should be filled with breast tissue.

◊ Baby's nose and chin should rest lightly on your breast.

◊ The deeper the latch, the better for you and for baby!

If you've tried this process over and over with no luck, the next step is to look for issues that may be preventing baby from latching well.

Refer to pages 146 to 147 to learn more about lip and tongue-ties. If a lip or tongue-tie is keeping baby from taking in enough of your breast or from creating a good seal around your breast, this could be the cause of their improper latch. Consult your IBCLC to confirm your suspicions and talk to your pediatrician about having the tie released.

WHAT TO DO TO HEAL SORE NIPPLES:

◊ Experiment with different breastfeeding positions to see if another feels better.

◊ Using different breastfeeding positions helps switch up where baby is applying the most suction, so you're not constantly experiencing damage to the same spot.

◊ Frequently (approximately every 15 minutes) express drops of breast milk and dab it on your nipples. Studies show that breast milk is more effective at healing than both nipple creams and lanolin.

◊ If breastfeeding is too painful, pump and bottle-feed until you can get help.

It's worth trying to pinpoint what's causing you pain when breastfeeding. When a baby latches improperly over a period of time, your milk supply can decrease, and you can get plugged ducts and milk blisters. Fighting through the pain won't prevent any of that from happening.

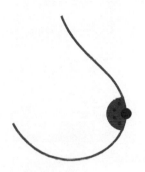

EVERTED NIPPLE
· Stays everted (has
  significant shape
  or definition)

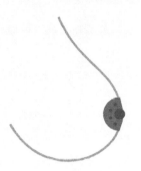

FLAT NIPPLE
· No (or very little)
  eversion

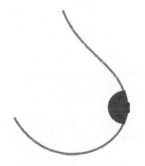

PSUEDO-INVERTED NIPPLE
· Everts with stimulation

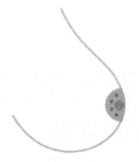

INVERTED NIPPLE
· Does not evert with
  stimulation

I HAVE A COLD/THE FLU/ FOOD POISONING!

DIAGNOSTICS: Germs, spoiled food

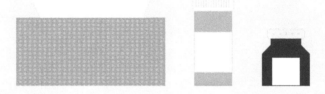

If you're sick, hang in there, take care of yourself, and keep breastfeeding if you can. Being sick doesn't necessarily mean that you need to quarantine yourself. It's very, very rare for a mom to need to stop feeding due to her illness. Most common illnesses, including the flu, are fine and it's even encouraged to keep breastfeeding through them.

When it comes to your baby, continuing to breastfeed is the best thing to do because your baby was exposed before you even knew you were sick, and (fun fact) your milk now has specialized antibodies to help protect baby against whatever germs made you ill. Yes, your body is that amazing.

Of course, be sure to tell your doctor that you're breastfeeding in case you need medication.

TROUBLESHOOTING TIPS

- Rest! Rest! Rest!
- Stay hydrated, both for your health and to protect your milk supply.
- Take extra vitamin C.
- Many medications are compatible with breast-feeding. They are ranked from L1 to L5. A lactation consultant can look up specific medications for you, or you can download the Mommy Meds app.
- Many cold symptoms can be treated with natural remedies. For more information, visit https://kelly mom.com/bf/can-i-breastfeed/meds/cold-remedy/.

Remember to ask for help and lighten your load as much as possible when you're sick. Breastfeed while in bed in the side-lying position and work hard to get enough fluids. Breast milk supply can dip while you're sick if you don't get enough fluids, and some medications can compound this.

If baby does get sick, it's just as important to keep breastfeeding them. If they are having trouble latching or staying on your breast because of congestion, try suction-ing their nose or using a saline nasal spray to clear their nasal passages.

CODE 006:

MY BACK AND SHOULDERS KILL ME WHEN I BREASTFEED!

<u>DIAGNOSTICS</u>: Leaning into baby, not using support

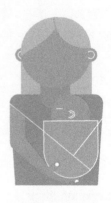

Postpartum back and shoulder pain can make many aspects of life with a baby challenging. You're already carrying baby everywhere, sometimes in heavy car seats, and you may be lugging around a diaper bag that rivals Mary Poppins's bag. It's wise to actively try to prevent poor posture and to be sure you're not weighing yourself down with too much when carrying baby's essentials.

This is another reason it's important to listen to your body. If you're uncomfortable in a certain breastfeeding position or when carrying baby in their car seat, take note. Your body is relying on you to take care of yourself just as well as you take care of baby.

TROUBLESHOOTING TIPS

- ◊ There's no right or wrong when it comes to breast-feeding positions. The right position is the one that is comfortable for you and baby and allows baby to effectively transfer milk.

- ◊ In the first few days after birth, the cross-cradle and football positions are most common. The cross-cradle allows you to latch baby deeply and keep them in a deep latch throughout the feed. Use whatever hold you can execute properly without causing yourself pain or discomfort.

- ◊ Remember not to lean into baby while nursing, but to instead bring them to your breast.

- ◊ Try applying a heating pad to your back, neck, and shoulders while breastfeeding or between sessions.

- ◊ Ask your partner or support person to massage the areas that hurt.

- ◊ Consider going to a massage therapist or chiropractor.

Sometimes back and shoulder pain just happens, even if you're mindful of your posture and breastfeeding positions. Remember that your body may also be sore immediately after having your baby simply from the act of giving birth.

CODE 007:

MY BREASTS ARE CRAZY SWOLLEN!

DIAGNOSTICS: (Normal) breast milk transitioning around day three to five

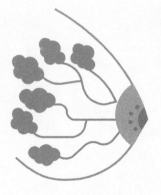

Whoa, momma! If your breasts look and feel like cantaloupes (basketballs, even?), they are probably not feeling too great. This is a relatively short but sometimes painful phase.

Your milk came in, which is awesome. Now, you need to help your body figure out how much milk it really needs to produce so you're not dealing with an oversupply.

As you're trying to relieve the pain of engorgement, be careful not to send your body mixed messages. The immediate relief of a full pumping session can tell your body to keep making too much milk, and the cycle will continue.

TROUBLESHOOTING TIPS

◊ Do not use pumping or heat as your primary means of relieving engorgement. This will compound the issue and make your breasts fuller and more uncomfortable over time.

◊ Apply cold compresses (bags of frozen peas or corn) to your breast tissue for 15 minutes, a couple of times an hour.

◊ Continue feeding baby on demand.

◊ Avoid applying cold right before the feed.

◊ If you are so full that no milk will come out, apply a warm compress right before breastfeeding for a few minutes.

◊ If you are having a difficult time compressing your breasts because of fullness, apply reverse pressure softening right before latch. Place your index fingers at your areola, parallel to each other and positioned vertically with the nipple between them, and push toward your chest wall for a few seconds. Then, repeat with your fingers positioned horizontally. This pushes the fluid farther back into your breast and makes your breast more malleable.

◊ Initial engorgement should resolve in 24 to 48 hours. If it lasts longer, reach out to a lactation consultant.

Sometimes, the most frustrating side effect of engorgement can be that your breasts are too hard for baby to properly latch. Between the desire to relieve the pain and the frustration of getting baby to latch, be careful you're not allowing a poor latch.

Massage your breasts and express just enough milk to soften them and make a deep latch easier for baby. Also, try different breastfeeding positions. Never let baby continue to breastfeed when their latch is too shallow or you'll risk painful injury to your nipples. A proper latch—deep and wide—will also help baby draw more milk from your breasts.

Unresolved engorgement can lead to plugged ducts. Be sure to read up on the signs and symptoms and how to treat them on page 62.

MOM TO MOM

"You do NOT have to nurse in public. You can find a private room, sit in your car, sit on a toilet in a public restroom, sit under a table at a reception, etc. (I've done all of those!) If your modesty and privacy are important to you, then honor that. There is absolutely nothing wrong with not wanting to breastfeed in public, so do not feel as if you have to place yourself in an uncomfortable position that feels wrong to you. Your body, your choice."

— Amy, Little Rock, AR

CODE 008:

HELP, MY MILK HASN'T COME IN!

DIAGNOSTICS: (Normal) if it's day one to five, you have colostrum

Keep in mind that everybody and every body is different. When you begin to panic that you don't feel like your milk has come in, ask yourself a few questions:

AM I BASING THIS ON SOMEONE ELSE'S EXPERIENCE?

Not all breasts get as full as others or follow the same schedule.

HAVE I BEEN PUTTING BABY TO MY BREAST FREQUENTLY, AT LEAST 8 TO 12 TIMES IN 24 HOURS?

Remember that your body needs to be told how much milk to make. The more baby latches and breastfeeds, the more milk your body will produce.

AM I STILL PRODUCING COLOSTRUM?

Breast milk production starts with colostrum, and that's what your breasts will produce for three to five days following birth. Remind yourself that baby's tummy is still very small at this age and they only need a small amount of colostrum at each feeding.

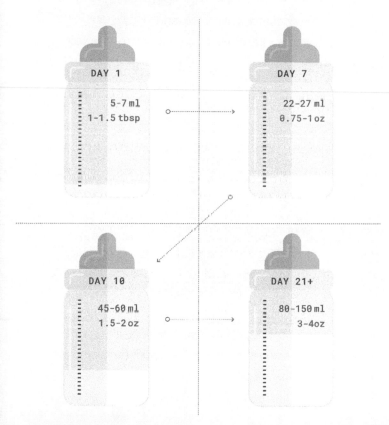

DAY 1
5-7 ml
1-1.5 tbsp

DAY 7
22-27 ml
0.75-1 oz

DAY 10
45-60 ml
1.5-2 oz

DAY 21+
80-150 ml
3-4 oz

TROUBLESHOOTING TIPS

◌ For the first three to five days you will have colostrum, which is highly concentrated, specialized breast milk full of nutrients and antibodies intended for your baby at this time.

◌ It's rich in protein, which helps stabilize baby's blood sugar, acts as a laxative, and seals baby's GI tract so it's less permeable to infection for the rest of their life!

◌ A full serving of colostrum is 2 to 10 milliliters.

◌ Around day three to five, your milk will transition, volume will increase, and your breasts may feel fuller.

◌ If you don't think your milk has transitioned by day five, reach out to a lactation consultant.

If baby is producing enough wet and dirty diapers, and they seem satisfied after breastfeeding, try not to worry if you're within that five-day window when your body is still producing colostrum. You do not need to supplement with formula if your pediatrician hasn't asked you to. If after five days you are still concerned that your milk hasn't transitioned, get in touch with your OB-GYN or midwife and a lactation consultant.

MOM TO MOM

"Ask for help. Don't expect that because breastfeeding is natural it will be easy. Never give up on your hardest day. Nurse your baby in public all you want because there's NOTHING shameful or wrong with it."

— Leah, Montpilier, VA

CODE 009:

CAN I EAT THAT?! HOW MUCH WATER DO I HAVE TO DRINK?

DIAGNOSTICS: Myths, not planning ahead or taking time to take care of yourself

Feeding yourself while breastfeeding should:

1. Absolutely be a priority

2. Not be complicated

Let's get this out of the way right here: You do not have to eliminate dairy or anything else from your diet unless you have a valid reason to believe you should.

Begin by simply feeding yourself. You will likely be very hungry in the first few days and weeks. Listen to your hunger. Also, do not forget to listen to your thirst. Dehydration can have a serious impact on your milk supply, so you should consider drinking water your part-time job, in addition to the full-time job that is breastfeeding a newborn.

What can you eat? Anything! Bonus points for foods that you can easily feed yourself with one hand. Stock your pantry and refrigerator with protein bars and other nutrition-packed snacks you can grab while on the go or when stuck under a napping baby.

TROUBLESHOOTING TIPS

- ◊ Although studies show moms need an additional 300 to 500 calories per day while breastfeeding (compared to pre-pregnancy diet), most moms accomplish this by eating to satiety and maintaining three meals plus a couple snacks each day.

- ◊ There should be no need to count calories.

- ◊ There isn't a specific diet you need to maintain while breastfeeding, and there's no list of foods you can't eat.

- ◊ Advice to not eat spicy or gassy foods is a myth

- ◊ Adequate hydration can usually be accomplished by drinking enough water to satisfy thirst.

- ◊ Most moms find they are very thirsty while breast-feeding or pumping, so keep a full water bottle nearby!

- ◊ Refer back to pages 58 to 59 for recommendations on what and how much to eat.

What about caffeine? One serving of caffeine per day (for example, one cup of coffee or one soda) is considered compatible with breastfeeding. Just keep in mind that fussi-ness may be correlated to a quad venti latte.

MY BABY ACTS LIKE THEY'RE STARVING!

DIAGNOSTICS: Normal

Babies can be so dramatic, am I right? You just fed them, and here they are, rooting and screaming their heads off, sucking on your partner's earlobe like it's a turkey leg. The thing to know about babies is that they need to eat a lot some days. All that growing is a high caloric expenditure for them.

You can get a feel for how much baby is successfully consuming by tracking wet and dirty diapers because what's coming out had to get in there in the first place. If all that seems normal and your breasts feel emptied and/or soft after you nurse, then you know baby is getting breast milk at each feeding.

The next logical conclusion is they are just plain hungry and it doesn't matter if you just fed them because, like hobbits, they expect breakfast, second breakfast, elevenses . . . and so on.

TROUBLESHOOTING TIPS

◊ Babies go through several growth spurts in the first year.

◊ There are four in the first six weeks, typically starting around days two to three and seven to 10, and weeks two to three and four to six.

◊ They can last a few days to a week.

◊ During growth spurts, babies will get lots of wet diapers.

◊ Growth spurts are are marked by increased fussiness, gas, cluster feeding (small feeds spaced close together; see CODE 011 on page 116), increased night feeding, and insistence on being held.

◊ Baby may also spit up more than usual.

◊ Continue to feed baby on demand, but be aware that baby may want to do lots of non-nutritive or comfort sucking. You should still expect 8 to 12 feeds every 24 hours.

◊ If you experience sore nipples or exhaustion, you can limit feeds to 20 to 25 minutes max and use breast massage and compression. That will help speed up breastfeeds and make milk transfer more efficient.

◊ Babywearing, skin-to-skin, infant gas drops, pacifiers, and pumping/bottle-feeding (if you've introduced bottles) can all help get you through these tough days.

◊ Plan for tough nights, tag-team with your partner, and bring in additional support if you can.

◊ If you suspect your baby is not getting enough milk, see your pediatrician or a lactation consultant.

MOM TO MOM

"Be kind to yourself! Drink way more water than you think you need and invest in a good bra. Also, ignore everyone who thinks they know better than you. You're the mom now."

— Maureen, Philadelphia, PA

MY BABY WON'T STOP SNACKING!

DIAGNOSTICS: Normal

Possibly one of the most frustrating experiences as a breastfeeding mother is wrapping up a long nursing session, handing baby off to your partner, and not even being able to get through eating a hot meal before baby is showing signs of hunger again.

The words "cluster feeding" can spark vivid memories of challenging nights for anyone who's had a child. Cluster feeding is when baby decides to nurse nearly back-to-back, usually in the evening. It's not indicative of a dip in your milk supply. Your baby got plenty of milk from you; they just want more.

If it feels like you aren't making enough milk when these cluster feedings begin, your body will adapt within a couple of days. Cluster feeding is one way baby tells your body that they will need more milk soon.

The upside to cluster feeding is most of the time baby is gearing up to get in a long stretch of sleep.

TROUBLESHOOTING TIPS

◊ Cluster feeding occurs most commonly in the late afternoon or evening and is often referred to as the "witching hour" (but can last two to four hours daily).

◊ Settle in on the couch and feed baby frequently. Don't forget to keep the TV remote and maybe your cell phone within arm's reach.

◊ Breast massage and breast compressions can help make feeds more efficient. While baby is nursing, support them with one hand, then use your other hand to encircle your breast, with your thumb on one side and fingers on the other. Gently squeeze and massage your breast, working your fingers from the top of your breast down toward your nipple, like squeezing toothpaste from a tube.

◊ If you're not up for the frequent snacking, a well-timed bottle can give you a break. (Don't forget to pump if baby gets a bottle.)

Cluster feeding can coincide with baby's fussy time of night, or when they're teething or not feeling well. The breastfeeding relationship is not strictly about giving your baby food; sometimes they're simply looking for comfort.

I THINK MY BABY IS ALLERGIC TO SOMETHING I'M EATING!

DIAGNOSTICS: Occurs in some babies

If baby is excessively fussy, and they have other symptoms like projectile vomit, cough, diarrhea, congestion, or a rash, there is a small possibility that your baby could have a food sensitivity or food allergy to something they're exposed to through your breast milk.

A very fussy baby who does not have any other symptoms is usually not dealing with a food sensitivity or allergy. Refer to page 32 to read more about gas and page 113 to read about growth spurts.

If you believe your baby may have a food sensitivity or allergy, it's important that you take them to your pediatrician. They can advise you on how to move forward safely for both you and baby. You may be able to target the food that's bothering baby and eliminate it from your diet.

TROUBLESHOOTING TIPS

◊ Signs of a sensitivity or allergy are inconsolable fussiness, pungent gas, and mucus or blood in baby's stool.

◊ If you notice one of these obvious reactions, alert your pediatrician. They may have you go on an elimination diet that will help pinpoint what is causing the reaction.

◊ Elimination diets are usually accompanied by scheduled stool samples at your pediatrician's office.

◊ Do not start an elimination diet without the guidance of your pediatrician or a lactation consultant.

Many moms of babies with allergies and sensitivities go on to successfully breastfeed after elimination diets. Sometimes, though, these diets can be challenging and cost-prohibitive. If elimination diets aren't a good fit for you or don't work for you, there are many nourishing formulas on the market free of the food your baby can't tolerate. The ultimate goal is to feed your baby, and there's more than one way to do that.

IT HURTS WHEN I PUMP!

DIAGNOSTICS: Low-quality breast pump, pumping too long, suction too high, flanges wrong size

We've already advised you not to tolerate pain while breast-feeding, and the same applies for pumping. If it hurts when you pump, something needs to be tweaked or changed entirely. You definitely don't want the pain to escalate to an injury. The good news is it should be relatively easy to diagnose the source of your discomfort and fix it.

TROUBLESHOOTING TIPS

◊ There is a big difference between low-quality and high-quality personal pumps. Look at reviews and research them in advance. Connect with a local lactation consultant and see which ones she likes. A low-quality pump can damage your nipples.

◊ The standard pump time is 15 to 20 minutes in place of a breastfeed or 10 minutes if you're pumping after a breastfeed. Don't "pump to empty." Follow the standard times.

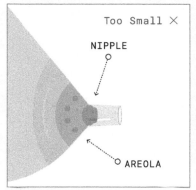

Too Small ✕

NIPPLE

AREOLA

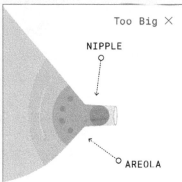

Too Big ✕

NIPPLE

AREOLA

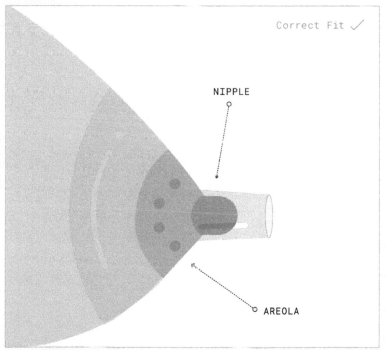

Correct Fit ✓

NIPPLE

AREOLA

◊ The suction (vacuum) should always be as high as you can comfortably go.

◊ When pumping, the flange should pull in your nipple and a little of your areola. Your nipple should move freely in the "tunnel" of the flange. If your nipple rubs against the sides of the tunnel, your flange is too small. If the tunnel pulls in a lot of areola, it's too big. The right flange will usually also be the one that feels the most comfortable.

◊ Some moms find putting coconut oil or nipple cream on the inside of the flange before pumping helps decrease the friction.

◊ Combining hand massage with pumping (hands-on pumping) can dramatically increase pumped volume.

Flanges are a great place to start. Remember that your nipples can change shape and size throughout your breastfeeding journey and what once fit could be too big or too small now. If you've checked that and everything else above and you're still experiencing pain, check in with your lactation consultant or medical provider. You may be dealing with vasospasms (contraction of the blood vessels) or a bleb (milk blister).

MOM TO MOM

"It's hard—ask for help! Watch other people breastfeed; it's weird to say, but we've lost that piece in our society and it's the best way to learn."

— Jessica, Honolulu, HI

CODE 014:

MY BABY WON'T TAKE FROZEN BREAST MILK!

DIAGNOSTICS: Excess lipase, broken bags, storage system

If baby is pushing their bottle away, spitting out milk, refusing to swallow, and generally not happy about what's in their bottle, they may not be cool with the way the milk tastes.

We know that bag of frozen breast milk is liquid gold and was the product of a lot of work and maybe some tears. It sucks when something is amiss with it once it's reheated. In some cases, though, it's salvageable. In others, it could be great for a baby milk bath, which moisturizes the skin and helps soothe diaper rash.

TROUBLESHOOTING TIPS

◊ Does your breast milk smell or taste soapy or stale when defrosted? It could have extra lipase, an enzyme that breaks down fat to help baby digest your milk. It's still safe to feed to baby. If baby refuses it, you can flash-scald future milk before freezing. To flash-scald, heat the breast milk in a pan to about 180°F or until tiny bubbles form around the edges but it hasn't reached a rolling boil. For the milk you've already frozen, you can try cutting it (after thawing) with freshly pumped milk to lessen the taste or adding one drop of alcohol-free vanilla extract.

- Does your breast milk smell or taste metallic or fishy? It could be chemical oxidation. Some people think drinking bottled water and lowering polyunsaturated fats in your diet can help. This milk is fine to give baby as well, as long as they don't mind.

- If milk smells sour or rotten, check the bag for holes or leaks. Look to see if it was tightly sealed. Make sure pumped milk smells normal before freezing it.

- Check the settings on your freezer and make sure your freezer is working properly.

- How long has the milk been frozen? Some moms find their milk does not stay good for six months. You may have milk that expires sooner.

Breast milk that is spoiled or rancid should go straight into the trash or down the drain. We are so sorry for your loss.

CODE 015:

MY BABY NEEDS FORMULA, TOO, AND I'M FREAKING OUT!

DIAGNOSTICS: Low milk supply, slow weight gain, food allergies, preference

Successful breastfeeding can include formula. Sometimes, adding formula to your feeding schedule can be the break you need to breastfeed longer. You should never, ever feel like you've failed at feeding your baby or parenting if you feed your baby formula.

Breastfeeding looks different for every family. For your family, that might mean "combo feeding," giving baby both breast milk and formula. Some moms combo-feed from the start, and some moms will exclusively breastfeed for a certain amount of time and then combo-feed when baby is older.

TROUBLESHOOTING TIPS

- ◊ Many people find that combo-feeding is what works best in their family. That's awesome!

- ◊ Keep in mind that although breast milk is the healthiest choice for most babies, it doesn't have to be "all or nothing."

○ Some moms exclusively breastfeed for the first few months and introduce some formula when they return to work. Breastfeeding can look different for each family.

○ Formula is more constipating, so watch baby's stooling pattern as you introduce it.

○ You may need to experiment with formulas to find the one that works best for your baby.

○ Some babies do better with soy or goat formula.

○ Breast milk and formula have different expiration times. Formula expires sooner, so any breast-milk-plus-formula bottle will need to be fed within the formula's time frame.

○ Your pediatrician can provide you with formula resources.

It's very important to remember that if you combine breast milk and formula in the same bottle, you should prepare the formula according to the directions separately, and then add breast milk to it. Never use your breast milk as a substitute for the water needed for formula powder or concentrated liquid formula. Never add powdered or concentrated formula to your breast milk.

UGH! I DON'T WANT ANYONE TO TOUCH ME!

DIAGNOSTICS: Exhaustion, growth spurt, high-needs baby

You just got done sharing your entire body with another person for nine-plus months, and now they spend half the day stuck to you. It is not unreasonable to want the time when baby is not breastfeeding (or needing comfort and closeness) to be a time when nobody else touches you. This can include pets, partners, and even your other children. You are not a bad mother or partner or person if you don't want to be kissed, hugged, or sat on when you're feeling like this.

It's helpful to be upfront about how you're feeling and why with the people in your life who may want to cuddle or snuggle. Explain that it's not personal—you still love them, but your body simply needs a break. In time, you'll be up for more touching and back to your old self. For now, you need to set some boundaries.

TROUBLESHOOTING TIPS

◊ Moms often report feeling "touched out" at the end of the day—especially on difficult days where they held a fussy baby the whole time. This is your body's normal physiological response to overstimulation.

◊ Practice self-care. Take a five-minute break. Walk outside and take a couple of deep breaths. Take a shower. Make yourself food. Call a friend. Do something intentional that feels restorative, even if you can squeeze in only a couple of minutes for yourself.

◊ Share your feelings with your partner, friends, and family.

◊ If your thoughts or feelings are concerning to you, consider talking to a professional.

◊ It's normal for baby to experience periods of extra fussiness. If it feels extreme, mention it to your pediatrician.

If you are feeling antsy or angry while holding and trying to console your fussy baby, it's okay to put baby down in a safe spot, like a crib, and walk away for a few minutes while you collect yourself or ask for someone else to take over.

CODE 017:

I DON'T HAVE ENOUGH MILK!

DIAGNOSTICS: Not removing breast milk
frequently, difficult delivery or start to
breastfeeding, various physical factors

Your milk supply can change based on a number of factors.
Stress, dehydration, and some medications can cause a dip
in your milk supply. Also, if you're away from baby and you
don't pump as frequently as you breastfeed or you don't
remove as much milk from your breasts as baby would, your
body will read that as a signal to produce less milk.

The good news is this is not permanent, and it's probably
not as bad as you think it is.

TROUBLESHOOTING TIPS

◊ Many moms have a "perceived low supply" because they are comparing themselves to other moms. Social media can make this even worse!

◊ If you are feeding your baby 8 to 12 times every 24 hours, feeds take approximately 25 minutes or less, and your baby gets at least four to six wet diapers daily and is gaining weight appropriately, then chances are you have a strong supply!

◊ If you suspect you have low supply, speak to your pediatrician or lactation consultant.

◊ If you do have low supply, there are ways to increase it. You may be given a plan that includes more feeding, pumping, herbs, changes in diet, or more efficient milk removal. Plans are very specific to each mom. It's definitely not one-size-fits-all, so seek out an expert's opinion.

One way to try to increase your supply without interventions or any special foods or herbs is to have a day with baby when your only tasks are to rest, drink as much water as possible, and get baby on your breast as frequently as they will let you. Make it a Netflix day!

MY BABY CHOKES WHEN WE BREASTFEED!

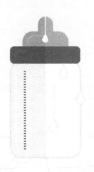

If low supply is a problem, oversupply is also not ideal, unfortunately. Yes, it's possible for your breasts to make too much milk. If you're thinking you can just pump out the extra to manage the situation, we regret to inform you that that just makes things worse. Remember that every time you remove milk from your breasts, via baby or pump, you're telling your body to make more. If you've already got too much, more is not what you need.

Oversupply can cause baby to choke or gulp quickly, causing them to take in air, which leads to gas (see page 32). It can also make baby clamp down on your nipple in an effort to stop or slow the flow, which can lead to pain and nipple damage.

TROUBLESHOOTING TIPS

○ For some moms, their super-strong supply comes with a downside: a flow that's difficult for baby to handle. This is common in the first six weeks and during the morning feeds.

○ If you feel super full, you can hand-express or pump just enough to take the edge off the first let-down before bringing baby to breast.

○ Try positioning baby at an angle so their head is higher than their bottom. This position will give baby more control over the flow.

○ Try "laid-back breastfeeding." This position also gives baby more control.

○ Time helps. Your supply should regulate around six weeks, and it will probably settle on a volume and flow that is more manageable for baby.

○ Keep a towel or blanket handy while nursing to clean up excess milk that may spray when baby unlatches.

After your milk transitions, be sure baby is emptying your breast before offering them the other side. Don't switch sides before your breast feels empty.

MY BABY WON'T SLEEP!

<u>DIAGNOSTICS</u>: Growth spurt, normal sleep pattern, teething, developmental leap, illness, change in environment

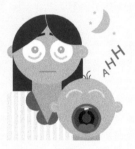

We don't always sleep when baby sleeps (and we wouldn't be sad if people stopped doling out that advice like it's the cure for new-parent exhaustion), but we certainly need that time to rest, recover, and get other stuff done. So when baby isn't sleeping, it can feel like an urgent and stressful situation.

Like all newborn challenges, this phase will pass, but knowing that still doesn't make it much easier when you are living it. Try to ease up on your obligations so that when baby does sleep you can actually try to catch up on whatever you need to do. And know that it's okay to feel frustrated by this, but that there are ways to work through it.

TROUBLESHOOTING TIPS

- ◊ Set realistic expectations. Babies are often more alert at night in the first six weeks. During growth spurts, babies feed frequently at night. It's very normal for breastfed babies under a year to still wake up a couple of times a night.

- ◊ If you're considering a sleep coach, work with one who is "breastfeeding friendly." Sleep coaches will typically work with you once baby is 16 weeks and 16 pounds. Even if baby is sleeping longer, you may still need to pump to maintain your supply.

- ◊ Encourage cluster feeding in the late afternoon or evening. Babies may do that to "tank up" for the night.

- ◊ Make sure you have a consistent nighttime routine, which will signal to baby that it's time to start winding down.

- ◊ Teething, illness, developmental leaps, vacation, or any change in routine can affect baby's sleep.

- ◊ Don't compare your baby to other babies. All babies have different temperaments and sleep patterns.

CAN I GIVE MY BABY A PACIFIER ALREADY?!

DIAGNOSTICS: High suck need, growth spurts

Pacifiers can be a godsend. They can also be controversial. This is one of those choices that only a parent can make based on the information they've armed themselves with, what's best for their family, and what they feel is best for their baby.

Pacifier use in the first days and weeks of baby's life can affect breastfeeding if it masks baby's hunger cues and takes place at times when baby should be on your breast to signal your body to make milk. If you feel like you can offer baby a pacifier and be mindful that it should not be a substitute for your breast, it's possible to introduce one right away.

If you'd rather wait until your milk is in and breastfeeding is going well, you can try introducing a pacifier after three to four weeks. The American Academy of Pediatrics recommends offering a pacifier for naps and nighttime to help prevent SIDS. Please don't freak out if baby won't take a pacifier; although some babies love pacifiers, some strongly dislike them from the very beginning. They are each their own little person, after all. It may help if you try a few different pacifier brands. You may find that baby has a favorite shape or style of pacifier and will only take that one.

TROUBLESHOOTING TIPS

- Some babies have a very high suck need. All babies have a high suck need during growth spurts.

- It's not generally advised to give baby a pacifier (or any artificial nipple) before four weeks.

- There may be times where a pacifier can be part of the plan early on.

- If you've recently introduced a pacifier, watch to make sure it's not covering baby's hunger cues.

- Most lactation consultants prefer pacifiers that are closer to the shape of mom's nipple (not orthodontic).

- Whether to introduce a pacifier is a question that can evoke strong opinions. Do what feels right for your family!

MY BABY WON'T TAKE A BOTTLE!

DIAGNOSTICS: Not introduced in the appropriate window, not given frequently enough, teething

So you're scheduled to head back to the office in less than a month, and you just discovered your baby refuses to take a bottle from you. Don't panic! They can smell your fear. I mean, for real—babies pick up on your stress, and that's not going to help any of this.

Stay calm. First, have you left the room—or the house even—and had another caregiver try to bottle-feed baby? It could be they simply don't want you to give them a bottle because they know the real deal is right there. They're looking at them. Try having your partner take on this task.

If that doesn't work right away, try different styles of nipples and bottles. There are many bottles and nipples on the market that closely resemble a breast. Remember, you'll also want the flow of the nipple to be slower. Learn more about paced bottle-feeding on page 150.

Try warming the milk (but don't make it too hot). You can even warm the nipple by running it under warm water.

If your baby has a preferred breastfeeding hold, replicate that with the bottle. Or maybe they associate that hold with receiving a breast, so try a new hold.

The key is patience and persistence, and sometimes someone else's help.

TROUBLESHOOTING TIPS

◊ Ideally, the bottle should be introduced between weeks four and six and, once introduced, given approximately once daily to keep baby used to it.

◊ Make sure you're giving an appropriate amount of milk. The average size of a breast milk bottle from three weeks on is 3 ounces. (Fun fact: Breast milk changes as baby gets older in terms of fat and caloric content, but the volume stays the same!)

◊ Teething can cause baby to refuse a bottle. Has baby been drooling? Lots of hands in mouth? If so, try teething remedies or numbing their gums right before a feed.

◊ Did baby take a bottle previously but won't now? Offer a bottle frequently as a snack, when baby is tired, and while walking or bouncing baby. Sometimes, changing the brand of the bottle you're using makes a difference.

I HAVE NO IDEA HOW TO INTRODUCE SOLIDS!

DIAGNOSTICS: Lacks current information

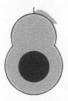 Once you get into the breastfeeding flow, it can become so easy to feed baby breast milk that adding solids, while an exciting new milestone, can feel like a lot of work. There's no need to overcomplicate this. You can and should introduce solids gradually, and some of the best first foods require very minimal prep.

Some families prefer to start out giving their babies mashed and puréed foods, and others like to do baby-led weaning. Baby-led weaning is a method of giving baby whole, mashed-up foods that they feed themselves. Baby-led weaning fans say this method lets babies explore food and self-pace their intake. It's also as simple as it gets. You just give baby the food you're already eating. You'll need to make sure to cut the food into safe sizes, so pick up a book on baby-led weaning and talk to your pediatrician for guidance on adding solids to your child's diet.

TROUBLESHOOTING TIPS

- Most pediatricians recommend starting solids around six months, once the baby is showing signs of readiness.

- Signs of readiness include:
  - Baby can sit up without support.
  - Baby has lost the tongue-thrust reflex.
  - Baby is developing the "pincer" grasp.
  - Baby is interested in solids.

- Start with one "meal" (a few bites) and work your way up to three meals and two snacks by one year.

- If you start around six months, food does not need to be puréed. Most babies will do well with smashed-up foods like avocado and sweet potato.

- Avoiding sweet foods so baby doesn't prefer sweets is a myth. Breast milk is sweet!

- Introduction of new foods should be spaced out by two to three days, so potential allergies can be identified.

- Solids are a complement to breast milk for babies under a year. Breastfeed baby before offering solids. One hour after breastfeeding is the perfect time to offer solids.

- Don't be discouraged if baby isn't excited about solids. They are all on their own schedule!

OWWWW! I FEEL A PAINFUL KNOT IN MY BREAST!

DIAGNOSTICS: Oversupply, going too long without pumping or breastfeeding, tight clothes, pressure on one area of breast, cracked or open tissue

As much as it can hurt, you have to get to work treating a plugged duct as soon as you notice it. Don't take a chance on it escalating to mastitis by hoping it will work its way out. This is one of those situations that gets worse before it gets better in terms of pain. Working out a plugged duct is not comfortable. Heat plus massage is the magic combo. Locate the knot and massage it directly with your thumb. You can do this while taking a shower or in a hot bath. Go at it for a minute or two, as long as you can stand it, then give yourself a break and try hand-expressing milk between massages.

Another technique is to submerge the affected breast in a bowl of warm water with a half cup of plain Epsom salts for 10 minutes. While submerged, massage the affected area toward the nipple. Follow with suction (either baby or pump).

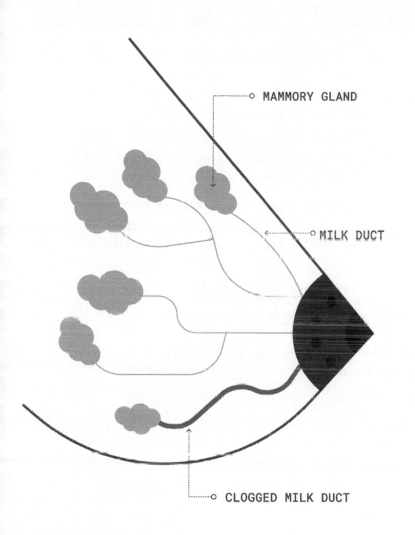

MAMMORY GLAND

MILK DUCT

CLOGGED MILK DUCT

TROUBLESHOOTING TIPS

◊ A plugged duct usually first appears as a tender, hard spot in the breast, and it quickly becomes more painful. If it's not cleared within one or two days, it can become mastitis (breast infection).

◊ Clearing the plug is a manual process of massaging it to break it up and move it out either via the nipple or up through the lymph node in the armpit.

◊ Don't knock it until you try it: Many moms swear by using a vibrator to massage the plug and break it up. You can also try a very strong hand massager.

◊ For recurrent plugged ducts, taking sunflower lecithin daily may reduce their frequency.

◊ If you have a stubborn plug that won't clear, some women's physical therapy centers offer ultrasound therapy and massage therapists who will work it out for you.

◊ If you're not able to clear the plug, it may turn into mastitis. One of the first signs of mastitis is a fever and chills. If you've had a fever for 24 hours, you'll need an antibiotic prescription from your OB-GYN.

MOM TO MOM

"Give yourself grace and remember it's a learning experience. Ask for help, there is no need to suffer."

— Aryn, Decatur, IL

WHEN BABY FEEDS, IT FEELS LIKE CRUSHED GLASS OR SANDPAPER ON MY NIPPLES!

DIAGNOSTICS: Tongue-tie

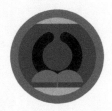

It's not normal for your nipples to bleed or for you to feel intense pain. It's not something to power through. If it's a tongue-tie, there's a path to relief!

Some signs of a lip or tongue-tie include:

◊ Baby is not able to latch for a long period or not latching deeply.

◊ Baby is not gaining enough weight and/or seems to nurse constantly.

◊ Mom's nipple starts looking like the wedge end of a tube of lipstick after baby comes off the breast, sometimes accompanied by a compression stripe across the tip.

You can also look inside baby's mouth to see if you notice what looks like a lip or tongue-tie. Refer to the diagram on page 157. If you see anything concerning, reach out to a lactation consultant.

TROUBLESHOOTING TIPS

- ○ If breastfeeding is still painful beyond the second week or your nipples are extremely damaged or sore, it's time to seek professional help. Contact a local lactation consultant. She will evaluate your baby and the breastfeed to see if the issue is correctable by technique. If not, she'll recommend an ear, nose, and throat doctor or a dentist in your area who specializes in diagnosing and releasing tongue-ties. A thorough evaluation and recommendation from professionals with expertise in this area is the best place to start

- ○ If your baby is diagnosed with a tongue-tie, it means that their lingual frenulum, that little fold of tissue under the tongue, is limiting baby's full range of motion, making breastfeeding difficult for baby and painful for you. Some parents opt to have a "release," which typically restores full range of motion.

- ○ Many babies who have tongue-ties also have upper lip ties. Upper lip ties are when baby's labial (lip) frenulum is tight. This prevents baby from being able to flange their lip like a fish and may add to breastfeeding difficulties.

WILL GIVING MY BABY A BOTTLE RUIN BREASTFEEDING?

DIAGNOSTICS: Returning to work, mom needs a break, sore nipples, date night

Bottle-feeding can work for all mother-baby relationships. Even mothers who don't work outside the home or exclusively feed their babies breast milk can find freedom in giving baby a bottle or getting someone else to bottle-feed baby.

Paced bottle-feeding is ideal for breastfed babies and recommended by the American Academy of Pediatrics. This gives you more control over baby's intake (of either breast milk or formula), and it helps reduce the amount of air they take in, which can lead to gassy discomfort. It also mimics the flow of milk from the breast and can keep baby from becoming accustomed to the faster flow of milk from a bottle, which could lead them to getting frustrated at the breast.

TROUBLESHOOTING TIPS

1. Hold baby in a more upright or semi-reclined position. Avoid feeding baby a bottle while they are lying flat.

2. Position the bottle horizontally, not upside down. You want just enough milk to fill the nipple.

3. Encourage baby to latch on the bottle nipple as they would your breast. Instead of inserting the nipple into their mouth, tickle their lips and nose with it and get them to latch on instead.

4. Be sure their lips are flanged around the bottle nipple just like you'd want them to be around your nipple.

5. Allow baby to take their time, and plan to bottle-feed for about the same amount of time they'd be at your breast.

6. You can slow down and manage baby's pace by switching sides, just like you'd switch breasts.

7. Burping baby after each ounce they drink also helps slow the pace and gives baby time to determine when they are full.

8. Don't try to get baby to eat more than they need just to finish off a bottle. Once baby shows signs of satiety, put the bottle aside and burp them.

PACED BOTTLE-FEEDING TIPS:

◊ Be sure that other caregivers are following this same approach.

◊ When you are beginning to figure out how many ounces baby may want to take from a bottle, prepare smaller amounts of milk so you don't risk wasting what's left over (especially breast milk) when they don't finish the whole bottle. Reminder: 3 ounces of breast milk in a bottle is a full feed from three weeks on.

◊ Just as you would feed based on baby's hunger cues (page 23), look out for signs that they are full to know when to stop: not showing that they want more after breaks, drowsing off, pushing the bottle away, letting milk dribble out of their mouth instead of swallowing it.

MOM TO MOM

"Remember that both the nursing and bottle feeding bonds are incredible, and that your mental health is just as crucial to the conversation about when to nurse or stop nursing."

— Rita, Charlotte, NC

CODE 026:

BABY WON'T BREASTFEED AT ALL!

DIAGNOSTICS: Frequent bottles in early weeks, fast bottles, too much milk in bottles, teething, illness, not breastfeeding frequently enough

Technology has given us a lot of great advances, but it has yet to give us a bottle that fully replicates a breast. Bottles are not the devil. They are, at minimum, helpful to have, and for many they are a necessity. It's understandable that many families choose to introduce bottle-feeding into a breastfed baby's life. One drawback, though, is that early and frequent bottle-feeding could cause baby to lose interest in receiving milk from a breast.

If this happens, try not to worry, but seek help from a lactation consultant. You can work to adopt the paced bottle-feeding techniques outlined on page 149. Stay calm, patient, and persistent.

TROUBLESHOOTING TIPS

- The most common reason that babies reject the breast is because they are receiving many bottles and the flow is too fast. The paced bottle-feeding technique dramatically improves the chances that baby will be able to go back and forth between bottle and breast.

- Babies who get used to large feeds and fast flow will have a harder time at the breast. Around three weeks, baby's average daily intake plateaus at 25 ounces per day. The average breast milk bottle is three ounces— and it stays at three ounces. (Phew! You don't need to make more and more milk as baby gets older!)

- Try offering the breast at every feed. Offer it when baby is sleepy and try partway through the bottle-feed. Offer it as a snack between bottles.

- Try having a "babymoon," where you take the baby to bed for a day or two, spending as much time lying together as possible and offering the breast.

- Is baby drooling? Lots of hands in mouth? Try treating their gums for teething discomfort.

- Don't give up. Although nursing strikes happen, babies rarely self-wean before a year. As long as you are persistent, baby will most likely return to your breast.

MY BABY SCREAMS, ARCHES THEIR BACK, AND CRIES FREQUENTLY AFTER FEEDING!

DIAGNOSTICS: Medical diagnosis

Call it colic, call it gas, but whatever it is, it's so hard to watch and it's exhausting. When your baby is inconsolable for long periods of time on a regular basis, it can really wear down everyone in the family. This is definitely something to see a medical professional about.

It's possible there is a real medical issue at play, and it could be something—like reflux—that can be helped with medication or modifying how you feed them. Sometimes, though, this period of intense, regular crying is something baby has to outgrow, and all you can do is try your best to comfort them. You should also balance that with taking care of yourself. Ask for help if you can so that you're not the only person trying to soothe your baby every night.

TROUBLESHOOTING TIPS

◊ Most babies are full, satiated, and relaxed after breastfeeds. If your baby arches and cries instead, mention it to your pediatrician.

◊ Some babies with reflux will spit up excessively, and some won't (silent reflux).

◊ If you suspect your baby has reflux, try feeding in "gravitational positions" with their head higher than their bottom. This will allow milk to settle in baby's tummy during the feed, instead of stomach acid being regurgitated into their esophagus.

◊ End each feed by holding baby upright on your chest for 10 to 15 minutes to allow the milk more time to settle.

◊ Babies who have reflux tend to dislike being laid flat, so try putting everything at a slight angle (changing pad, etc.) to see if that makes baby more comfortable.

◊ Reflux symptoms can mirror other feeding issues like oversupply and food sensitivities. Seek the help of a professional to work through the possibilities.

MY BREAST HAS AN ITCHY RASH, AND BABY HAS A THICK WHITE COATING ON THEIR TONGUE!

DIAGNOSTICS: Fungal infection, medical diagnosis

Does baby have a white patch on their tongue or inside their cheeks that you can't wipe away? Are your nipples itchy, red, and shiny? Thrush is very contagious and you and baby may be passing it back and forth to each other. This means that in order to curb this unpleasant shared yeast infection, you and baby will have to be treated at the same time, even if one of you is not showing signs of thrush yet. (Given time, it will pop up.)

Thrush can be persistent, so you have to be consistent with treatment, which can include a topical antifungal cream for your nipples, an oral gel for baby's mouth, and sometimes gentian violet—a messy, bright purple topical ointment—for your nipples and inside baby's mouth.

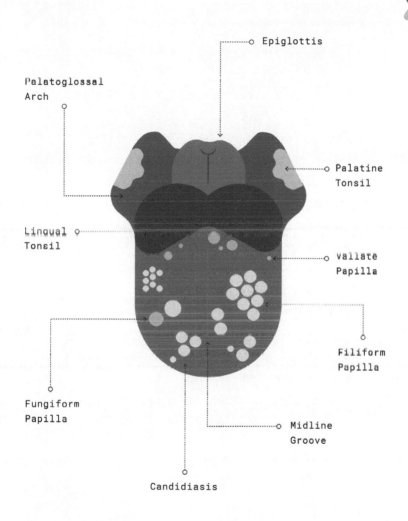

Epiglottis

Palatoglossal
Arch

Palatine
Tonsil

Lingual
Tonsil

Vallate
Papilla

Filiform
Papilla

Fungiform
Papilla

Midline
Groove

Candidiasis

TROUBLESHOOTING TIPS

◊ Thrush is a fungal infection that both mom and baby can get and pass back and forth.

◊ It can appear on mom's nipples, inside of baby's cheeks and tongue, and as a diaper rash.

◊ When mom has thrush on her nipples, it usually burns and feels very itchy. You usually see pink, flaky skin around the nipple and areola.

◊ On baby, it can appear as thick patches on the tongue and on the inside of their cheeks that won't easily wipe off.

◊ Most of the time thrush needs to be treated with an antifungal prescription. And it is most effective when mom and baby are treated simultaneously.

◊ Mom must also regularly boil and replace anything that comes into contact with the breast or baby's mouth during treatment.

◊ Thrush can be persistent and difficult to resolve.

MOM TO MOM

"Relax. Success or failure does
not hinge on this one aspect
of mothering. Don't let yourself
be in pain unnecessarily."

— Amy, Champaign, IL

CODE 029:

MY BABY JUST BIT MY BOOB!

<u>DIAGNOSTICS</u>: Teething, boredom, playing

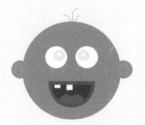

Biting is something many breastfeeding parents dread, but not all babies bite. And if they do, it's not necessarily going to become a regular thing.

Baby is learning and exploring. They are getting to know what their body does, like clenching their jaw shut. They are exploring the texture of your breasts. This exploratory phase can be considerably painful for you, though, especially if baby has or is in the process of cutting their tiny, razor-sharp teeth.

TROUBLESHOOTING TIPS

◊ The most common reason a baby bites is because they are teething. Try teething remedies and numbing the gums right before the feed.

◊ Typically, a bite happens at the end of the feed. Baby has to retract their tongue to bite down, so watch for that movement and pop them off the breast before they can bite you!

○ Don't make a game out of it. Babies are sensitive to mom's tone. You want to communicate "that hurt mommy," and "that's not okay," and end the feed. You can resume the feeding a little later if needed.

○ This is typically a short phase. Babies who bite while nursing most often only do it once or twice, so hang in there.

It probably feels counterintuitive, but if baby bites and won't let go, pull them into your breast instead of away from you. First, you don't want to pull baby off the nipple while they are still clamped on and latched. That's going to make it worse. Second, this will surprise baby. They don't want your boob shoved in their face, and they will unlatch to move their head out of the way. Don't hold them there more than a second. The point is to surprise them, not to prevent them from breathing.

CODE 030:

I DON'T KNOW HOW TO WEAN!

DIAGNOSTICS: End of nursing

The end of a breastfeeding relationship can come with a variety of feelings: sadness, anxiety, happiness, relief. They are all valid. Whatever the reason is that you feel you need to wean, there's more than one way to approach it.

TROUBLESHOOTING TIPS

◊ There are three types of weaning: baby-led weaning, parent-led weaning, and emergency weaning.

◊ Baby-led weaning is when baby decides when and how to wean. Breastfeeds will be eliminated naturally and easily over time as baby decides to supplement those calories with solid food. These babies will often breastfeed for two to four years or longer.

◊ Parent-led weaning is when mom encourages baby to drop breastfeeds or breast milk bottles, and she slowly brings down her supply. This can take four to eight weeks or more and should be done under the supervision of a lactation consultant. The more gradual the wean, the easier it is on mom and baby.

◊ Emergency weaning is when a mom must quickly wean for medical or personal reasons such as deployment or medical interventions. This should also be done under the supervision of a lactation consultant as this method puts mom at much higher risk for plugged ducts and mastitis.

It doesn't matter if you wean your baby at three weeks, three months, or three years. You did a great job breast-feeding, and you should be proud of yourself. You will, no doubt, continue feeding baby adequately and comforting them regularly. It's okay to feel sad about the end of this journey, and it's also okay to feel happy about it.

REFERENCES

KELLYMOM.COM

- www.kellymom.com/ages/newborn/nb-challenges/wean-shield/
- www.kellymom.com/bf/can-i-breastfeed/lifestyle/smoking/
- www.kellymom.com/ages/older-infant/fertility/
- www.kellymom.com/tandem-faq/04mom nutrition/
- www.kellymom.com/parenting/parenting-faq/gassybaby/
- www.kellymom.com/health/baby-health/food-sensitivity/

LA LECHE LEAGUE

- www.llli.org/breastfeeding-info/positioning/
- www.llli.org/breastfeeding-info/oversupply/
- www.llli.org/breastfeeding-info/tongue-lip-ties/
- www.llli.org/breastfeeding-info/thrush/

THIFTY NIFTY MOMMY

- www.thriftyniftymommy.com/do-it-yourself-easy-breastfeeding/

MOTHER LOVE

- www.motherlove.com/blogs/all/feeding-breastmilk
  -by-bottle-learn-paced-feeding-to-avoid-over
  feeding-your-baby
- www.motherlove.com/blogs/all/is-pumping-causing
  -you-pain

MEDELA

- www.medela.com/breastfeeding/mums-journey
  /storing-and-thawing-breast-milk

AMERICANPREGNANCY.ORG

- www.americanpregnancy.org/breastfeeding
  /breastfeeding-while-pregnant/

VERY WELL FAMILY

- www.verywellfamily.com/can-you-mix-breast
  -milk-and-infant-formula-431969

HEALTHY CHILDREN

- www.healthychildren.org/English/ages-stages
  /baby/sleep/Pages/Preventing-SIDS.aspx

ASKDRSEARS.COM

◊ www.askdrsears.com/topics/feeding-eating/breast
feeding/faqs/getting-baby-to-take-bottle

BABYLEDWEANING.COM

◊ www.babyledweaning.com/some-tips-to-get
-you-started/

RESOURCES

WEBSITES

AMERICAN ACADEMY OF PEDIATRICS

www.healthychildren.org/English/ages-stages/baby/breast
feeding/Pages/default.aspx

BREASTFEEDING AFTER BREAST AND NIPPLE SURGERIES

www.bfar.org/index.shtml

DR. JACK NEWMAN

Dr. Newman is a Canadian pediatrician and one of the leading experts in breastfeeding. You can find great videos and
fact sheets on his website.

www.breastfeedinginc.ca/

DR. SEARS

Dr. Sears is a respected pediatrician and breastfeeding expert.

www.askdrsears.com/topics/feeding-eating/breastfeeding

FMLA

www.dol.gov/general/topic/benefits-leave/fmla

KELLYMOM

Evidence-based breastfeeding information. This should be your first stop!

www.kellymom.com

LA LECHE LEAGUE

This is a nonprofit organization providing advocacy and education for breastfeeding. There is a lot of great information on their website, where you can also find your local La Leche League chapter.

www.lllusa.org

MARCH OF DIMES

English: www.marchofdimes.org/baby/the-nicu-family -support-program.aspx

Spanish: nacersano.marchofdimes.org/

NATIONAL WOMEN'S LAW CENTER TOOLKITS

www.nwlc.org/sites/default/files/pdfs/final_nwlcbreast feedingtoolkit2014_edit.pdf

NATIONAL WOMEN'S LAW CENTER FACT SHEET

nwlc-ciw49tixgw5lbab.stackpathdns.com/wp-content /uploads/2016/12Breastfeeding-Benefits-FS-4.pdf

PATIENT PROTECTION AND AFFORDABLE CARE ACT (ACA)
www.congress.gov/bill/111th-congress/house-bill/3590

POSTPARTUM RESOURCES FOR PARTNERS
www.postpartum.net/get-help/family/tips-for-postpartum
-dads-and-partners/

POSTPARTUM WORKBOOK FOR SELF-CARE
www.lifewithbabyworkbook.com

SUPPORT GROUPS

There is no overemphasizing how valuable local breast-feeding support groups can be. They are usually free or low-cost, and there you'll find your village of advice, support, camaraderie, someone to text at 2 a.m., and possibly friends for life!

Places to look for support groups near you:

◊ Hospitals

◊ Lactation consultant offices

◊ Breastfeeding stores or boutiques

◊ Women's centers and collectives

BOOKS

Gaskin, Ina May, *Ina May's Guide to Breastfeeding: From the Nation's Leading Midwife*

Huggins, Kathleen, *The Nursing Mother's Companion: The Breastfeeding Book Mothers Trust, from Pregnancy Through Weaning*

Huggins, Kathleen, *The Nursing Mother's Guide to Weaning: How to Bring Breastfeeding to a Gentle Close, and How to Decide When the Time Is Right*

Mohrbacher, Nancy, and Kathleen Kendall-Tackett, *Breastfeeding Made Simple: Seven Natural Laws for Nursing Mothers*

Sears, Martha, and William Sears, *The Breastfeeding Book: Everything You Need to Know About Nursing Your Child from Birth Through Weaning*

INDEX

ACKNOWLEDGMENTS

I've been lifted up and surrounded by an incredible community for as long as I've breastfed my four babies. I want to thank my mom for being the first person to encourage and support my breastfeeding efforts, and my whole family for always being my cheerleaders. A HUGE thank-you to my husband, Scott, who has always been 100 percent on my side, no matter how I chose to feed our babies. He has always taken on as much work as he possibly can, especially in the newborn months, so that I can focus on my breastfeeding relationship with all four of them.

Thank you to Jessica Martin-Weber of TheLeakyBoob.com for being a trusted online resource and friend. So much of my breastfeeding success is also because of the powerful online community, including my amazing blog readers, who have given me thoughtful and encouraging advice over the years. I'm also so grateful they have shared so much of their own breastfeeding journeys and struggles with me. Their stories shaped a lot of this book.

Thank you to Chrisie for helping with this book. Your professional insight into the technicalities of breastfeeding helped this become the resource I hoped it would be. And a final thank-you to my editor Morgan Shanahan for her vision for this project. I'm so proud of what we created together.

—Jill Krause

I am so lucky to have a village of strong and wise women whom I constantly lean on, learn from, and laugh with. I am grateful for every one of you!

I want to thank my parents, Bill and Sharon, and my sister, Vickie, for always supporting me in every way. And to Maryssa and Alex for letting me "mother" them before I was actually a mom. My gratitude to my family is never-ending. My three amazing sons (my loves) Ben, Ethan, and Sam are the ones who led me to the work of supporting families and always encourage me to accomplish my goals. They give me gifts every day, and I'm beyond thankful for their love and support.

Thank you to Gini Baker and Karen Hatcher, who were my first IBCLC teachers and mentors. Thank you to my IBCLC students, who have taught me more than I could ever teach you and thank you to the many families who have allowed me into your lives at a very vulnerable time, to support you and your little ones. This work is truly a blessing.

Last, so many thank-you's to Jill Krause and our editor Morgan Shanahan. You both made this a fun and rewarding project! Thanks for being kind, insightful, and patient as I learned the ropes. This has been an amazing experience!

—Chrisie Rosenthal, IBCLC

ABOUT THE AUTHORS

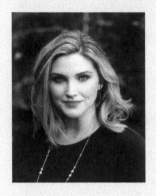 **JILL KRAUSE** is writer, photographer, and mother of four. Krause is an award-winning and internationally recognized blogger and content creator, and she has written about parenthood and pregnancy for over a decade at BabyRabies.com and now JillKrause.com. Her first published book, *50 Things to Do Before You Deliver: The First Time Mom's Pregnancy Guide*, was published in 2018. She is a graduate of the Missouri School of Journalism, University of Missouri, and lives outside of Austin with her husband, four kids, and two dogs. You can find her on Instagram at @Jillkraus.e.

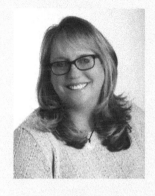 **CHRISIE ROSENTHAL** is a highly respected IBCLC (International Board Certified Lactation Consultant) and mom of three boys (including twins!) in Los Angeles. She is the founder of the Land of Milk and Mommy, a private practice supporting breastfeeding families. She also works for Cleo, a San Francisco startup that supports families from pregnancy through age five. She's a graduate from San Diego State University with a bachelors degree in Broadcasting and Film. You can reach out or learn more about her work at www.landofmilkandmommy.com.

Printed in the USA
CPSIA information can be obtained
at www.ICGtesting.com
CBHW040448310524
9306CB00013B/212